Acknowledgements

The collective knowledge generated from academic and applied research summarized in various references has been critical in the creation of this book which is best viewed as a comprehensive compilation and collection of information prepared by various official agencies which produce publications on dysphasia. Books in this series draw from various agencies and institutions associated with the United States Department of Health and Human Services, and in particular, the Office of the Secretary of Health and Human Services (OS), the Administration for Children and Families (ACF), the Administration on Aging (AOA), the Agency for Healthcare Research and Quality (AHRQ), the Agency for Toxic Substances and Disease Registry (ATSDR), the Centers for Disease Control and Prevention (CDC), the Food and Drug Administration (FDA), the Healthcare Financing Administration (HCFA), the Health Resources and Services Administration (HRSA), the Indian Health Service (IHS), the institutions of the National Institutes of Health (NIH), the Program Support Center (PSC), and the Substance Abuse and Mental Health Services Administration (SAMHSA). In addition to these sources, information gathered from the National Library of Medicine, the United States Patent Office, the European Union, and their related organizations has been invaluable in the creation of this book. Some of the work represented was financially supported by the Research and Development Committee at INSEAD. This support is gratefully acknowledged. Finally, special thanks are owed to Tiffany Freeman for her excellent editorial support.

DGAAM

DYSPHASIA

A MEDICAL DICTIONARY, BIBLIOGRAPHY,
AND ANNOTATED RESEARCH GUIDE TO
INTERNET REFERENCES

JAMES N. PARKER, M.D.
AND PHILIP M. PARKER, PH.D., EDITORS

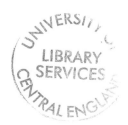

ii

ICON Health Publications
ICON Group International, Inc.
4370 La Jolla Village Drive, 4th Floor
San Diego, CA 92122 USA

Printed in the United States of America.

Last digit indicates print number: 10 9 8 7 6 4 5 3 2 1

Publisher, Health Care: Philip Parker, Ph.D.
Editor(s): James Parker, M.D., Philip Parker, Ph.D.

Publisher's note: The ideas, procedures, and suggestions contained in this book are not intended for the diagnosis or treatment of a health problem. As new medical or scientific information becomes available from academic and clinical research, recommended treatments and drug therapies may undergo changes. The authors, editors, and publisher have attempted to make the information in this book up to date and accurate in accord with accepted standards at the time of publication. The authors, editors, and publisher are not responsible for errors or omissions or for consequences from application of the book, and make no warranty, expressed or implied, in regard to the contents of this book. Any practice described in this book should be applied by the reader in accordance with professional standards of care used in regard to the unique circumstances that may apply in each situation. The reader is advised to always check product information (package inserts) for changes and new information regarding dosage and contraindications before prescribing any drug or pharmacological product. Caution is especially urged when using new or infrequently ordered drugs, herbal remedies, vitamins and supplements, alternative therapies, complementary therapies and medicines, and integrative medical treatments.

Cataloging-in-Publication Data

Parker, James N., 1961-
Parker, Philip M., 1960-

    Dysphasia: A Medical Dictionary, Bibliography, and Annotated Research Guide to Internet References / James N. Parker and Philip M. Parker, editors
          p.   cm.
    Includes bibliographical references, glossary, and index.
    ISBN: 0-497-00388-0
    1. Dysphasia-Popular works.   I. Title.

About the Editors

James N. Parker, M.D.

Dr. James N. Parker received his Bachelor of Science degree in Psychobiology from the University of California, Riverside and his M.D. from the University of California, San Diego. In addition to authoring numerous research publications, he has lectured at various academic institutions. Dr. Parker is the medical editor for health books by ICON Health Publications.

Philip M. Parker, Ph.D.

Philip M. Parker is the Eli Lilly Chair Professor of Innovation, Business and Society at INSEAD (Fontainebleau, France and Singapore). Dr. Parker has also been Professor at the University of California, San Diego and has taught courses at Harvard University, the Hong Kong University of Science and Technology, the Massachusetts Institute of Technology, Stanford University, and UCLA. Dr. Parker is the associate editor for ICON Health Publications.

About ICON Health Publications

To discover more about ICON Health Publications, simply check with your preferred online booksellers, including Barnes&Noble.com and Amazon.com which currently carry all of our titles. Or, feel free to contact us directly for bulk purchases or institutional discounts:

ICON Group International, Inc.
4370 La Jolla Village Drive, Fourth Floor
San Diego, CA 92122 USA
Fax: 858-546-4341
Web site: **www.icongrouponline.com/health**

Table of Contents

FORWARD

In March 2001, the National Institutes of Health issued the following warning: "The number of Web sites offering health-related resources grows every day. Many sites provide valuable information, while others may have information that is unreliable or misleading."[1] Furthermore, because of the rapid increase in Internet-based information, many hours can be wasted searching, selecting, and printing. Since only the smallest fraction of information dealing with dysphasia is indexed in search engines, such as **www.google.com** or others, a non-systematic approach to Internet research can be not only time consuming, but also incomplete. This book was created for medical professionals, students, and members of the general public who want to know as much as possible about dysphasia, using the most advanced research tools available and spending the least amount of time doing so.

In addition to offering a structured and comprehensive bibliography, the pages that follow will tell you where and how to find reliable information covering virtually all topics related to dysphasia, from the essentials to the most advanced areas of research. Public, academic, government, and peer-reviewed research studies are emphasized. Various abstracts are reproduced to give you some of the latest official information available to date on dysphasia. Abundant guidance is given on how to obtain free-of-charge primary research results via the Internet. **While this book focuses on the field of medicine, when some sources provide access to non-medical information relating to dysphasia, these are noted in the text.**

E-book and electronic versions of this book are fully interactive with each of the Internet sites mentioned (clicking on a hyperlink automatically opens your browser to the site indicated). If you are using the hard copy version of this book, you can access a cited Web site by typing the provided Web address directly into your Internet browser. You may find it useful to refer to synonyms or related terms when accessing these Internet databases. **NOTE:** At the time of publication, the Web addresses were functional. However, some links may fail due to URL address changes, which is a common occurrence on the Internet.

For readers unfamiliar with the Internet, detailed instructions are offered on how to access electronic resources. For readers unfamiliar with medical terminology, a comprehensive glossary is provided. For readers without access to Internet resources, a directory of medical libraries, that have or can locate references cited here, is given. We hope these resources will prove useful to the widest possible audience seeking information on dysphasia.

The Editors

---

[1] From the NIH, National Cancer Institute (NCI): **http://www.cancer.gov/cancerinfo/ten-things-to-know**.

CHAPTER 1. STUDIES ON DYSPHASIA

Overview

In this chapter, we will show you how to locate peer-reviewed references and studies on dysphasia.

The Combined Health Information Database

The Combined Health Information Database summarizes studies across numerous federal agencies. To limit your investigation to research studies and dysphasia, you will need to use the advanced search options. First, go to **http://chid.nih.gov/index.html**. From there, select the "Detailed Search" option (or go directly to that page with the following hyperlink: **http://chid.nih.gov/detail/detail.html**). The trick in extracting studies is found in the drop boxes at the bottom of the search page where "You may refine your search by." Select the dates and language you prefer, and the format option "Journal Article." At the top of the search form, select the number of records you would like to see (we recommend 100) and check the box to display "whole records." We recommend that you type "dysphasia" (or synonyms) into the "For these words:" box. Consider using the option "anywhere in record" to make your search as broad as possible. If you want to limit the search to only a particular field, such as the title of the journal, then select this option in the "Search in these fields" drop box. The following is what you can expect from this type of search:

- **Understanding Dysphagia: A Parent's Guide**

  Source: Exceptional Parent: 74-77. October 2002.

  Contact: Available from Exceptional Parent, 65 East Route 4, River Edge, NJ 07661. (201) 489-4111. Fax: (201) 489-0074. PRICE: $2.95 per online article.

  Summary: Parents need to be aware of the signs of swallowing problems (dysphagia) and know what to do if they suspect their child has a swallowing problem. This article provides parents with an overview of dysphagia, including types of swallowing problems, common signs of this condition, and the types of tests and procedures that take place when a child is evaluated. Parents are alerted to a list of common signs of dysphagia as well as the various tests that can be performed if further evaluation is necessary. If **dysphasia** is diagnosed, a plan of support should take the child's health and lifestyle into consideration. Relevant Web site addresses and contact information for supply resources also are provided.

- **Mandibular Resorption Due to Progressive Systemic Sclerosis: A Case Report**

  Source: Journal of Oral and Maxillofacial Surgery. 59(5): 565-567. May 2001.

  Contact: Available from W.B. Saunders Company. Periodicals Department, P.O. Box 629239, Orlando, FL 32862-8239. (800) 654-2452. Website: www.harcourthealth.com.

  Summary: Progressive systemic sclerosis (PSS), also known as scleroderma, is a connective tissue disorder of unknown origin, characterized by fibrosis of the skin and other visceral organs. The disease generally occurs between 30 and 50 years of age, and women are mostly affected. The disease progresses with the firmness of the skin leading to limitation of mobility of the fingers. The tight sclerotic skin causes extrinsic pressure and the overproduced collagen in the small arteries leads to the obliteration of the vessels and eventually induces destruction of the bone. This article reports a case of PSS with general and facial findings, and extensive mandibular (lower jaw) resorption. The patient, a 45 year old white woman, presented with a complaint of mobility of her anterior mandibular teeth. Her PSS had been diagnosed 21 years previously. The oral opening was reduced to 32 mm because of atrophy of the lip muscles and tightening of the skin. Intraoral examination revealed poor oral hygiene, loss of teeth, and periodontitis that was especially localized to the anterior mandibular region. After extensive evaluation, results revealed no other pathology, metabolic bone disease or neoplasia that could be causing her bone resorption. Esophageal involvement, with **dysphasia** (swallowing difficulty) and pulmonary (lung) involved were also diagnosed in this patient. 5 figures. 1 table. 18 references.

- **Esophageal Motility Disorders, Their Diagnosis and Management**

  Source: Practical Gastroenterology. 16(7): 13-14, 17, 21-22, 24-26. July-August 1992.

  Summary: The article explains that esophageal motility disorders are most commonly present with dysphagia for solids and liquids. Patients usually describe difficulty initiating a swallow (oropharyngeal dysphagia) or a sensation of food or liquid being hindered in its passage through the esophagus to the stomach (esophageal dysphagia). This article discusses the diagnosis and management of a group of disorders, including the multiple causes of oropharyngeal **dysphasia**, achalasia, spastic esophageal motility disorders, and scleroderma. For each disorder, the author also discusses the clinical presentation and recommends laboratory tests to confirm diagnosis. 2 figures. 3 tables. 10 references. (AA-M).

- **Developmental Language Disorders and Epilepsy**

  Source: Journal of Paediatrics and Child Health. 33(3): 277-280. June 1997.

  Contact: Available from Blackwell Science Pty Ltd. P.O. Box 378, Carlton, Victoria 3053, Australia. 61 3 9347 0300. Fax 61 3 9349 3016.

  Summary: This article reviews studies connecting developmental language disorders and epilepsy. The association of speech and language disorders with epilepsy is well known in children with acquired epileptic aphasia, involving such entities as Landau-Kleffner syndrome (LKS), continuous spike wave in slow wave sleep (CSWSS) epilepsy, and benign partial epilepsy with centro temporal spikes (BPECTS). The possible association between epilepsy and a subgroup of children with developmental **dysphasia** is reported less frequently. Lack of controlled prospective studies of sleep electroencephalograms (EEG), and the use of medication, in children with developmental dysphagia, may deny appropriate treatment strategies to children with severe developmental speech and language disorders. The authors recommend that before anti-epileptic medication is tried in individual children, limitations should be discussed with the parents: the treatment duration should be determined; goals should be set for continuation of therapy; pretreatment measures of speech and language should be carried out, including use of video records and standardized tests; the treatment should be at dosage levels used to control seizures; and there should be close monitoring for side effects. 1 table. 38 references.

Federally Funded Research on Dysphasia

The U.S. Government supports a variety of research studies relating to dysphasia. These studies are tracked by the Office of Extramural Research at the National Institutes of Health.[2] CRISP (Computerized Retrieval of Information on Scientific Projects) is a searchable database of federally funded biomedical research projects conducted at universities, hospitals, and other institutions.

Search the CRISP Web site at **http://crisp.cit.nih.gov/crisp/crisp_query.generate_screen**. You will have the option to perform targeted searches by various criteria, including geography, date, and topics related to dysphasia.

For most of the studies, the agencies reporting into CRISP provide summaries or abstracts. As opposed to clinical trial research using patients, many federally funded studies use animals or simulated models to explore dysphasia. The following is typical of the type of information found when searching the CRISP database for dysphasia:

- **Project Title: COORDINATION OF RESPIRATION AND DEGLUTITION**

  Principal Investigator & Institution: Perlman, Adrienne L.; Professor; Speech and Hearing Science; University of Illinois Urbana-Champaign Henry Administration Bldg Champaign, Il 61820

  Timing: Fiscal Year 2002; Project Start 15-JAN-2000; Project End 31-DEC-2003

  Summary: The close proximity of the larynx to the entrance of the esophagus, and the common pathway through the pharynx that both air and a swallowed bolus must traverse, require that swallowing and respiration be well coordinated. Discoordination can result in the aspiration of food, liquid, or oral secretions consequent risk of severe respiratory complications. Despite its critical function, the coordination of respiration with swallowing is not well-understood either in healthy individuals or in persons, such as stroke patients, who are known to be at high risk for developing aspiration pneumonia. Using respirodeglutometry, this research will characterize the joint timing of respiration with the swallow and simultaneously record respiratory airflow, submental surface electromyography, and swallow-associated acoustic signals. Two hundred forty normal subjects (120 male, 120 female) in five groups ranging from 3 to 85 years-of-age, and sixty medically stable stroke patients, will be studied. Respirodeglutometric (RDT) output will be digitized at 1000 samples/sec/channel

---

[2] Healthcare projects are funded by the National Institutes of Health (NIH), Substance Abuse and Mental Health Services (SAMHSA), Health Resources and Services Administration (HRSA), Food and Drug Administration (FDA), Centers for Disease Control and Prevention (CDCP), Agency for Healthcare Research and Quality (AHRQ), and Office of Assistant Secretary of Health (OASH).

while subjects swallow pre-measured 5, 10, and 15 ml volumes of water and pudding. For all subjects and for each swallow, the direction of respiration preceding and following the swallow, the duration of deglutition apnea, and five additional RDT temporal measures will be obtained. All stroke patients will also be seen for videofluoroscopic assessment within 24 hours of the RDT evaluation in order to directly assess the oral and pharyngeal stages of their swallow and to identify various indicators of dysphagia, including the presence/absence of laryngeal penetration and aspiration. Analysis will address i) effects of size and viscosity of swallowed material on timing of RDT measured events within the swallow, ii) changes in the coordination of respiration with swallowing in healthy subjects across the lifespan, iii) age and gender adjusted effects of stroke on such coordination, iv) adaptations of coordination by healthy subjects and stroke patients to feeding by a caregiver relative to self-feeding, and v) the relationship in stroke patients of videofluoroscopically- observed oropharyngeal **dysphasia** and aspiration to aberrant respiratory-swallowing patterns. Findings from this research can have a profound effect on patient evaluation procedures as well as on behavioral management techniques, clinical outcome goals, and medical costs for stroke patients.

Website: http://crisp.cit.nih.gov/crisp/Crisp_Query.Generate_Screen

- **Project Title: FUNCTIONAL PLASTICITY IN CHILDREN WITH HEMISPHERECTOMIES**

  Principal Investigator & Institution: Asarnow, Robert F.; Professor; None; University of California Los Angeles 10920 Wilshire Blvd., Suite 1200 Los Angeles, Ca 90024

  Timing: Fiscal Year 2002; Project Start 01-SEP-2000; Project End 31-AUG-2005

  Summary: This revised application addresses hypotheses developed from work that the investigators carried out in the initial UCLA Epilepsy Surgery Program concerning the extent and nature of functional plasticity in young children following early hemispherectomies. The proposed project addresses key questions concerning the capacity of the human brain for functional plasticity. The investigators will test hypotheses about the functional plasticity of language, certain cognitive functions, and social communication in a unique cohort of children who have received left or right hemispherectomies for medially intractable epilepsy prior to 10 years of age. They will attempt to better define the temporal "window" for functional plasticity. They will determine if age at seizure onset and age at surgery predict the extent to which children show functional plasticity for specific linguistic, cognitive, and social communication function. The effect of seizure etiology on functional plasticity will be examined by comparing 1) children with and without evidence of cortical **dysphasia** in the resected hemisphere and 2) children with Rasmussen encephalitis to children with cerebral infarcts within the non-cortical dysplasia groups. This project represents a singular opportunity to more fully integrate the work conducted in their respective laboratories in order to examine the interrelation between language, cognition, and social communication in the isolated right and left hemispheres of children receiving early hemispherectomies. These questions will be addressed at two, five and ten years of age in the UCLA Pediatric Epilepsy Surgery Program. The investigators are currently following almost 50 children starting from pre-surgical evaluation to follow-up intervals ranging from 1 to 12 years. During the follow-up evaluations, children will be administered a careful selected set of tasks which have been demonstrated in prior research to tap linguistic, cognitive and social communication function normally lateralized to either the left or right hemisphere. This will provide the investigators the opportunity to determine the extent to which an isolated left or right hemisphere can support functions normally supported by the resected hemisphere.

Website: http://crisp.cit.nih.gov/crisp/Crisp_Query.Generate_Screen

- **Project Title: THE NEURAL BASIS OF RATE CODING IN THE AUDITORY SYSTEM**

  Principal Investigator & Institution: Elliott, Taffeta M.; Ctr for Neurobiology Behavior; Columbia University Health Sciences Po Box 49 New York, Ny 10032

  Timing: Fiscal Year 2003; Project Start 01-SEP-2003; Project End 31-AUG-2005

  Summary: (provided by applicant): This research proposal aims to uncover how the auditory system codes rate as a feature of acoustic communication. Understanding human speech requires judgments based on rapid temporal intervals. A detailed consideration of how temporal processing detects linguistic contrasts will be important to understanding many disorders of language including **dysphasia** and dyslexia. Xenopus laevis provides a tractable model organism for this objective because of its rich repertoire of vocalizations that vary in the rate of repeated clicks. Tests of behavioral psychophysics will determine whether male clawed frogs categorically perceive the two female calls that differ only in click rate: one call signifies sexual receptivity of the female and stimulates male calling, whereas the other call functions as an antiaphrodisiac that suppresses male calling. Electrophysiological recording in the auditory midbrain and medulla will reveal whether cells are rate-tuned, and whether they form a spatial map of rate. Finally, neuroanatomical tracing will outline the construction of rate-sensitive auditory circuits and their influence on the control of vocal production.

  Website: http://crisp.cit.nih.gov/crisp/Crisp_Query.Generate_Screen

The National Library of Medicine: PubMed

One of the quickest and most comprehensive ways to find academic studies in both English and other languages is to use PubMed, maintained by the National Library of Medicine.[3] The advantage of PubMed over previously mentioned sources is that it covers a greater number of domestic and foreign references. It is also free to use. If the publisher has a Web site that offers full text of its journals, PubMed will provide links to that site, as well as to sites offering other related data. User registration, a subscription fee, or some other type of fee may be required to access the full text of articles in some journals.

To generate your own bibliography of studies dealing with dysphasia, simply go to the PubMed Web site at **http://www.ncbi.nlm.nih.gov/pubmed**. Type "dysphasia" (or synonyms) into the search box, and click "Go." The following is the type of output you can expect from PubMed for dysphasia (hyperlinks lead to article summaries):

---

[3] PubMed was developed by the National Center for Biotechnology Information (NCBI) at the National Library of Medicine (NLM) at the National Institutes of Health (NIH). The PubMed database was developed in conjunction with publishers of biomedical literature as a search tool for accessing literature citations and linking to full-text journal articles at Web sites of participating publishers. Publishers that participate in PubMed supply NLM with their citations electronically prior to or at the time of publication.

- **A 60-year-old man with expressive dysphasia.**
  Author(s): McAndrew NA, Charles TJ.
  Source: Postgraduate Medical Journal. 1999 July; 75(885): 431-2.
  http://www.ncbi.nlm.nih.gov/entrez/query.fcgi?cmd=Retrieve&db=pubmed&dopt=Abstract&list_uids=10474733

- **A child with abnormal features and expressive dysphasia.**
  Author(s): Kumar RK, Nagi SP.
  Source: European Journal of Pediatrics. 2000 January-February; 159(1-2): 119-20.
  http://www.ncbi.nlm.nih.gov/entrez/query.fcgi?cmd=Retrieve&db=pubmed&dopt=Abstract&list_uids=10653345

- **A computational account of deep dysphasia: evidence from a single case study.**
  Author(s): Martin N, Saffran EM.
  Source: Brain and Language. 1992 August; 43(2): 240-74.
  http://www.ncbi.nlm.nih.gov/entrez/query.fcgi?cmd=Retrieve&db=pubmed&dopt=Abstract&list_uids=1393522

- **A new approach to the treatment of severe dysphasia: a case study.**
  Author(s): Davies CL, Grunwell P.
  Source: Br J Disord Commun. 1975 October; 10(2): 142-8. No Abstract Available.
  http://www.ncbi.nlm.nih.gov/entrez/query.fcgi?cmd=Retrieve&db=pubmed&dopt=Abstract&list_uids=1191508

- **A nucleus vocabulary in the therapy of dysphasia: word finding, naming and recall--case report.**
  Author(s): Stewart FJ.
  Source: Journal of the American Geriatrics Society. 1966 July; 14(7): 768-71.
  http://www.ncbi.nlm.nih.gov/entrez/query.fcgi?cmd=Retrieve&db=pubmed&dopt=Abstract&list_uids=5938738

- **A psychomotor approach to improving speech by modulating suprasegmental control in motor dysphasia and articulatory apraxia.**
  Author(s): Hadar U, Twiston-Davies R, Steiner TJ, Rose FC.
  Source: Adv Neurol. 1984; 42: 337-51. No Abstract Available.
  http://www.ncbi.nlm.nih.gov/entrez/query.fcgi?cmd=Retrieve&db=pubmed&dopt=Abstract&list_uids=6507181

- **Abnormal frequency mismatch negativity in mentally retarded children and in children with developmental dysphasia.**
  Author(s): Holopainen IE, Korpilahti P, Juottonen K, Lang H, Sillanpaa M.
  Source: Journal of Child Neurology. 1998 April; 13(4): 178-83.
  http://www.ncbi.nlm.nih.gov/entrez/query.fcgi?cmd=Retrieve&db=pubmed&dopt=Abstract&list_uids=9568762

- **Acute dysphasia associated with hypoglycemia.**
  Author(s): Raz I, Gotlieb D, Bar-On H.
  Source: Isr J Med Sci. 1984 August; 20(8): 729-30. No Abstract Available.
  http://www.ncbi.nlm.nih.gov/entrez/query.fcgi?cmd=Retrieve&db=pubmed&dopt=Abstract&list_uids=6469599

- **An elderly man with dysphasia and pyrexia.**
  Author(s): Jolobe OM.
  Source: Postgraduate Medical Journal. 1999 October; 75(888): 639.
  http://www.ncbi.nlm.nih.gov/entrez/query.fcgi?cmd=Retrieve&db=pubmed&dopt=A
  bstract&list_uids=10621919

- **An elderly man with dysphasia and pyrexia.**
  Author(s): Sathi N, Shinton RA.
  Source: Postgraduate Medical Journal. 1999 May; 75(883): 307-8.
  http://www.ncbi.nlm.nih.gov/entrez/query.fcgi?cmd=Retrieve&db=pubmed&dopt=A
  bstract&list_uids=10533643

- **An experimental study in dysphasia. An interim report.**
  Author(s): Wirz SL, Stanton JB.
  Source: Br J Disord Commun. 1968 April; 3(1): 66-74. No Abstract Available.
  http://www.ncbi.nlm.nih.gov/entrez/query.fcgi?cmd=Retrieve&db=pubmed&dopt=A
  bstract&list_uids=5665926

- **Anger associated with dysphasia.**
  Author(s): Fisher CM.
  Source: Trans Am Neurol Assoc. 1970; 95: 240-2. No Abstract Available.
  http://www.ncbi.nlm.nih.gov/entrez/query.fcgi?cmd=Retrieve&db=pubmed&dopt=A
  bstract&list_uids=5514380

- **Assessing everyday memory in patients with dysphasia.**
  Author(s): Cockburn J, Wilson B, Baddeley A, Hiorns R.
  Source: The British Journal of Clinical Psychology / the British Psychological Society.
  1990 November; 29 (Pt 4): 353-60.
  http://www.ncbi.nlm.nih.gov/entrez/query.fcgi?cmd=Retrieve&db=pubmed&dopt=A
  bstract&list_uids=2289071

- **Asynchronous language acquisition in developmental dysphasia.**
  Author(s): Ouellet C, Cohen H, Le Normand MT, Braun C.
  Source: Brain and Cognition. 2000 June-August; 43(1-3): 352-7.
  http://www.ncbi.nlm.nih.gov/entrez/query.fcgi?cmd=Retrieve&db=pubmed&dopt=A
  bstract&list_uids=10857724

- **Attenuated auditory event-related potential (mismatch negativity) in children with
  developmental dysphasia.**
  Author(s): Holopainen IE, Korpilahti P, Juottonen K, Lang H, Sillanpaa M.
  Source: Neuropediatrics. 1997 October; 28(5): 253-6.
  http://www.ncbi.nlm.nih.gov/entrez/query.fcgi?cmd=Retrieve&db=pubmed&dopt=A
  bstract&list_uids=9413003

- **Atypical dominance for language in developmental dysphasia.**
  Author(s): Martins IP, Antunes NL, Castro-Caldas A, Antunes JL.
  Source: Developmental Medicine and Child Neurology. 1995 January; 37(1): 85-90.
  http://www.ncbi.nlm.nih.gov/entrez/query.fcgi?cmd=Retrieve&db=pubmed&dopt=A
  bstract&list_uids=7530220

- **Autism and receptive dysphasia: evaluation of comparative studies.**
  Author(s): von Tetzchner S, Martinsen H.
  Source: Scandinavian Journal of Psychology. 1981; 22(4): 283-96.
  http://www.ncbi.nlm.nih.gov/entrez/query.fcgi?cmd=Retrieve&db=pubmed&dopt=Abstract&list_uids=7336175

- **Bilateral intracarotid amytal injection. A study of dysphasia, disturbance of consciousness and paresis.**
  Author(s): Hommes OR, Panhuysen LH.
  Source: Psychiatr Neurol Neurochir. 1970 November-December; 73(6): 447-59. No Abstract Available.
  http://www.ncbi.nlm.nih.gov/entrez/query.fcgi?cmd=Retrieve&db=pubmed&dopt=Abstract&list_uids=5531971

- **Category specific access dysphasia.**
  Author(s): Warrington EK, McCarthy R.
  Source: Brain; a Journal of Neurology. 1983 December; 106 (Pt 4): 859-78.
  http://www.ncbi.nlm.nih.gov/entrez/query.fcgi?cmd=Retrieve&db=pubmed&dopt=Abstract&list_uids=6652466

- **Causes and management of dysphasia.**
  Author(s): Hovard L.
  Source: Br J Hosp Med. 1992 September 16-October 6; 48(6): 320-4. Review.
  http://www.ncbi.nlm.nih.gov/entrez/query.fcgi?cmd=Retrieve&db=pubmed&dopt=Abstract&list_uids=1422547

- **Cerebellar hypoperfusion and developmental dysphasia in a male.**
  Author(s): Oki J, Takahashi S, Miyamoto A, Tachibana Y.
  Source: Pediatric Neurology. 1999 October; 21(4): 745-8. Review.
  http://www.ncbi.nlm.nih.gov/entrez/query.fcgi?cmd=Retrieve&db=pubmed&dopt=Abstract&list_uids=10580890

- **Clinical studies on Chinese multilinguals with dysphasia.**
  Author(s): Tan CT, Rapport RL.
  Source: Singapore Med J. 1981 June; 22(3): 140-3. No Abstract Available.
  http://www.ncbi.nlm.nih.gov/entrez/query.fcgi?cmd=Retrieve&db=pubmed&dopt=Abstract&list_uids=7302620

- **Comparative trial of volunteer and professional treatments of dysphasia after stroke.**
  Author(s): Meikle M, Wechsler E, Tupper A, Benenson M, Butler J, Mulhall D, Stern G.
  Source: British Medical Journal. 1979 July 14; 2(6182): 87-9.
  http://www.ncbi.nlm.nih.gov/entrez/query.fcgi?cmd=Retrieve&db=pubmed&dopt=Abstract&list_uids=466329

- **Comprehension and production of idioms in dysphasia.**
  Author(s): Bush PG, Drummond SS.
  Source: Archives of Physical Medicine and Rehabilitation. 1985 October; 66(10): 697-700.
  http://www.ncbi.nlm.nih.gov/entrez/query.fcgi?cmd=Retrieve&db=pubmed&dopt=Abstract&list_uids=2413823

- **Computerised augmentative communication devices for people with dysphasia: design and evaluation.**
  Author(s): Rostron A, Ward S, Plant R.
  Source: Eur J Disord Commun. 1996; 31(1): 11-30.
  http://www.ncbi.nlm.nih.gov/entrez/query.fcgi?cmd=Retrieve&db=pubmed&dopt=Abstract&list_uids=8776429

- **Confusion, dysphasia, and asterixis following metrizamide myelography.**
  Author(s): Smith MS, Laguna JF.
  Source: The Canadian Journal of Neurological Sciences. Le Journal Canadien Des Sciences Neurologiques. 1980 November; 7(4): 309-11.
  http://www.ncbi.nlm.nih.gov/entrez/query.fcgi?cmd=Retrieve&db=pubmed&dopt=Abstract&list_uids=7214247

- **Deep dysphasia in a case of phonemic deafness: role of the right hemisphere in auditory language comprehension.**
  Author(s): Duhamel JR, Poncet M.
  Source: Neuropsychologia. 1986; 24(6): 769-79.
  http://www.ncbi.nlm.nih.gov/entrez/query.fcgi?cmd=Retrieve&db=pubmed&dopt=Abstract&list_uids=3808285

- **Deep dysphasia: an analog of deep dyslexia in the auditory modality.**
  Author(s): Michel F, Andreewsky E.
  Source: Brain and Language. 1983 March; 18(2): 212-23.
  http://www.ncbi.nlm.nih.gov/entrez/query.fcgi?cmd=Retrieve&db=pubmed&dopt=Abstract&list_uids=6188511

- **Deep dysphasia: analysis of a rare form of repetition disorder.**
  Author(s): Katz RB, Goodglass H.
  Source: Brain and Language. 1990 July; 39(1): 153-85.
  http://www.ncbi.nlm.nih.gov/entrez/query.fcgi?cmd=Retrieve&db=pubmed&dopt=Abstract&list_uids=2207619

- **Development dysphasia and electroencephalographic abnormalities.**
  Author(s): Maccario M, Hefferen SJ, Keblusek SJ, Lipinski KA.
  Source: Developmental Medicine and Child Neurology. 1982 April; 24(2): 141-55.
  http://www.ncbi.nlm.nih.gov/entrez/query.fcgi?cmd=Retrieve&db=pubmed&dopt=Abstract&list_uids=6178637

- **Developmental dysphasia: clinical importance and underlying neurological causes.**
  Author(s): Njiokiktjien C.
  Source: Acta Paedopsychiatr. 1990; 53(2): 126-37. Review.
  http://www.ncbi.nlm.nih.gov/entrez/query.fcgi?cmd=Retrieve&db=pubmed&dopt=Abstract&list_uids=1704678

- **Developmental dysphasia: relation between acoustic processing deficits and verbal processing.**
  Author(s): Tallal P, Stark RE, Kallman C, Mellits D.
  Source: Neuropsychologia. 1980; 18(3): 273-84.
  http://www.ncbi.nlm.nih.gov/entrez/query.fcgi?cmd=Retrieve&db=pubmed&dopt=Abstract&list_uids=6158017

- **Differentiating the language disorder in dementia from dysphasia--the potential of a screening test.**
  Author(s): Stevens SJ.
  Source: Eur J Disord Commun. 1992; 27(4): 275-88.
  http://www.ncbi.nlm.nih.gov/entrez/query.fcgi?cmd=Retrieve&db=pubmed&dopt=Abstract&list_uids=1285000

- **Dysphasia accompanied by periodic lateralized epileptiform discharges.**
  Author(s): Ono S, Chida K, Fukaya N, Yoshihashi H, Takasu T.
  Source: Intern Med. 1997 January; 36(1): 59-61.
  http://www.ncbi.nlm.nih.gov/entrez/query.fcgi?cmd=Retrieve&db=pubmed&dopt=Abstract&list_uids=9058104

- **Dysphasia and constructional dyspraxia items, and Wechsler Verbal and Performance IQs in retardates.**
  Author(s): Davis LJ Jr, Reitan RM.
  Source: Am J Ment Defic. 1967 January; 71(4): 604-8. No Abstract Available.
  http://www.ncbi.nlm.nih.gov/entrez/query.fcgi?cmd=Retrieve&db=pubmed&dopt=Abstract&list_uids=6033120

- **Dysphasia and dementia in residential homes.**
  Author(s): Ames D.
  Source: Age and Ageing. 1990 November; 19(6): 426-7.
  http://www.ncbi.nlm.nih.gov/entrez/query.fcgi?cmd=Retrieve&db=pubmed&dopt=Abstract&list_uids=1704681

- **Dysphasia during sleep due to an unusual vascular lesion.**
  Author(s): Harrison MJ.
  Source: Journal of Neurology, Neurosurgery, and Psychiatry. 1981 August; 44(8): 739.
  http://www.ncbi.nlm.nih.gov/entrez/query.fcgi?cmd=Retrieve&db=pubmed&dopt=Abstract&list_uids=7299412

- **Dysphasia, dyspraxia, and dysarthria: distinguishing features, Part I.**
  Author(s): Boss BJ.
  Source: J Neurosurg Nurs. 1984 June; 16(3): 151-60. No Abstract Available.
  http://www.ncbi.nlm.nih.gov/entrez/query.fcgi?cmd=Retrieve&db=pubmed&dopt=Abstract&list_uids=6564142

- **Dysphasia, dyspraxia, and dysarthria: distinguishing features, Part II.**
  Author(s): Boss BJ.
  Source: J Neurosurg Nurs. 1984 August; 16(4): 211-6. No Abstract Available.
  http://www.ncbi.nlm.nih.gov/entrez/query.fcgi?cmd=Retrieve&db=pubmed&dopt=Abstract&list_uids=6565751

- **Dysphasia. A review of recent progress.**
  Author(s): Wyke M.
  Source: British Medical Bulletin. 1971 September; 27(3): 211-7. Review.
  http://www.ncbi.nlm.nih.gov/entrez/query.fcgi?cmd=Retrieve&db=pubmed&dopt=Abstract&list_uids=4937263

- **Dysphasia: the patient, his family, and the nurse.**
  Author(s): Buck M.
  Source: Cardiovasc Nurs. 1970 September-October; 6(5): 51-6. No Abstract Available.
  http://www.ncbi.nlm.nih.gov/entrez/query.fcgi?cmd=Retrieve&db=pubmed&dopt=Abstract&list_uids=5202180

- **EEG changes and epilepsy in developmental dysphasia.**
  Author(s): Dlouha O, Nevsimalova S.
  Source: Suppl Clin Neurophysiol. 2000; 53: 271-4. No Abstract Available.
  http://www.ncbi.nlm.nih.gov/entrez/query.fcgi?cmd=Retrieve&db=pubmed&dopt=Abstract&list_uids=12741009

- **Effect of stimulus context and response coding variables on word retrieval performances in dysphasia.**
  Author(s): Dunn ND, Russell SS, Drummond SS.
  Source: Journal of Communication Disorders. 1989 June; 22(3): 209-23.
  http://www.ncbi.nlm.nih.gov/entrez/query.fcgi?cmd=Retrieve&db=pubmed&dopt=Abstract&list_uids=2738193

- **Effects of localised cerebral lesions and dysphasia on verbal memory.**
  Author(s): Coughlan AK.
  Source: Journal of Neurology, Neurosurgery, and Psychiatry. 1979 October; 42(10): 914-23.
  http://www.ncbi.nlm.nih.gov/entrez/query.fcgi?cmd=Retrieve&db=pubmed&dopt=Abstract&list_uids=556517

- **Expressive dysphasia possibly related to FK506 in two liver transplant recipients.**
  Author(s): Reyes J, Gayowski T, Fung J, Todo S, Alessiani M, Starzl TE.
  Source: Transplantation. 1990 December; 50(6): 1043-5.
  http://www.ncbi.nlm.nih.gov/entrez/query.fcgi?cmd=Retrieve&db=pubmed&dopt=Abstract&list_uids=1701571

- **Expressive dysphasia presenting as psychiatric disorder--a case report.**
  Author(s): Gangat AE, Cernochova V.
  Source: South African Medical Journal. Suid-Afrikaanse Tydskrif Vir Geneeskunde. 1997 September; 87(9): 1150.
  http://www.ncbi.nlm.nih.gov/entrez/query.fcgi?cmd=Retrieve&db=pubmed&dopt=Abstract&list_uids=9358840

- **Focal cerebral hypoperfusion in children with dysphasia and/or attention deficit disorder.**
  Author(s): Lou HC, Henriksen L, Bruhn P.
  Source: Archives of Neurology. 1984 August; 41(8): 825-9.
  http://www.ncbi.nlm.nih.gov/entrez/query.fcgi?cmd=Retrieve&db=pubmed&dopt=Abstract&list_uids=6331818

- **From conceptual intention to utterance: a study of impaired language output in a child with developmental dysphasia.**
  Author(s): Chiat S, Hirson A.
  Source: Br J Disord Commun. 1987 April; 22(1): 37-64. No Abstract Available.
  http://www.ncbi.nlm.nih.gov/entrez/query.fcgi?cmd=Retrieve&db=pubmed&dopt=Abstract&list_uids=2445369

- **Genetic basis of developmental dysphasia. Report of eleven familial cases in six families.**
  Author(s): Billard C, Toutain A, Loisel ML, Gillet P, Barthez MA, Maheut J.
  Source: Genet Couns. 1994; 5(1): 23-33.
  http://www.ncbi.nlm.nih.gov/entrez/query.fcgi?cmd=Retrieve&db=pubmed&dopt=Abstract&list_uids=8031532

- **Gliclazide-induced hepatitis, hemiplegia and dysphasia in a suicide attempt.**
  Author(s): Caksen H, Kendirci M, Tutus A, Uzum K, Kurtoglu S.
  Source: J Pediatr Endocrinol Metab. 2001 September-October; 14(8): 1157-9.
  http://www.ncbi.nlm.nih.gov/entrez/query.fcgi?cmd=Retrieve&db=pubmed&dopt=Abstract&list_uids=11592575

- **Guidelines for rehabilitating stroke patients. 1. Dysphasia--and the nurse.**
  Author(s): Brocklehurst JC.
  Source: Nurs Mirror Midwives J. 1971 October 22; 133(17): 17-9. No Abstract Available.
  http://www.ncbi.nlm.nih.gov/entrez/query.fcgi?cmd=Retrieve&db=pubmed&dopt=Abstract&list_uids=5209992

- **Hand signals for dysphasia.**
  Author(s): Eagleson HM Jr, Vaughn GR, Knudson AB.
  Source: Archives of Physical Medicine and Rehabilitation. 1970 February; 51(2): 111-3.
  http://www.ncbi.nlm.nih.gov/entrez/query.fcgi?cmd=Retrieve&db=pubmed&dopt=Abstract&list_uids=5437124

- **Hemispheric specialization using SPECT and stimulation tasks in children with dysphasia and dystrophia.**
  Author(s): Chiron C, Pinton F, Masure MC, Duvelleroy-Hommet C, Leon F, Billard C.
  Source: Developmental Medicine and Child Neurology. 1999 August; 41(8): 512-20.
  http://www.ncbi.nlm.nih.gov/entrez/query.fcgi?cmd=Retrieve&db=pubmed&dopt=Abstract&list_uids=10479040

- **Increased amplitude of the auditory P2 and P3b components in adolescents with developmental dysphasia.**
  Author(s): Adams J, Courchesne E, Elmasian R, Lincoln A.
  Source: Electroencephalogr Clin Neurophysiol Suppl. 1987; 40: 577-83. No Abstract Available.
  http://www.ncbi.nlm.nih.gov/entrez/query.fcgi?cmd=Retrieve&db=pubmed&dopt=Abstract&list_uids=2446852

- **Infantile autism and developmental receptive dysphasia: a comparative follow-up into middle childhood.**
  Author(s): Cantwell DP, Baker L, Rutter M, Mawhood L.
  Source: Journal of Autism and Developmental Disorders. 1989 March; 19(1): 19-31.
  http://www.ncbi.nlm.nih.gov/entrez/query.fcgi?cmd=Retrieve&db=pubmed&dopt=Abstract&list_uids=2708301

- **Language and intelligence in dysphasia: are they related?**
  Author(s): Edwards S, Ellams J, Thompson J.
  Source: Br J Disord Commun. 1976 October; 11(2): 83-97. No Abstract Available.
  http://www.ncbi.nlm.nih.gov/entrez/query.fcgi?cmd=Retrieve&db=pubmed&dopt=Abstract&list_uids=974011

- **Learning in dysphasia.**
  Author(s): Ettlinger G, Moffett AM.
  Source: Neuropsychologia. 1970 November; 8(4): 465-74.
  http://www.ncbi.nlm.nih.gov/entrez/query.fcgi?cmd=Retrieve&db=pubmed&dopt=Abstract&list_uids=5522573

- **Left hemiplegia without dysphasia, associated with congenitally absent right forearm.**
  Author(s): Hays P.
  Source: The British Journal of Psychiatry; the Journal of Mental Science. 1967 August; 113(501): 921.
  http://www.ncbi.nlm.nih.gov/entrez/query.fcgi?cmd=Retrieve&db=pubmed&dopt=Abstract&list_uids=6057666

- **Left thalamic hemorrhage with dysphasia: a report of five cases.**
  Author(s): Reynolds AF, Turner PT, Harris AB, Ojemann GA, Davis LE.
  Source: Brain and Language. 1979 January; 7(1): 62-73.
  http://www.ncbi.nlm.nih.gov/entrez/query.fcgi?cmd=Retrieve&db=pubmed&dopt=Abstract&list_uids=312127

- **Linguistic description in nonfluent dysphasia: utilization of pictograms.**
  Author(s): Cherepski MA, Drummond SS.
  Source: Brain and Language. 1987 March; 30(2): 285-304.
  http://www.ncbi.nlm.nih.gov/entrez/query.fcgi?cmd=Retrieve&db=pubmed&dopt=Abstract&list_uids=3567551

- **Medical pathology conference. Headache, fever, abnormal behavior, and dysphasia in an elderly man.**
  Author(s): Garcia JH, Sekar BC, Whitley RJ.
  Source: Ala J Med Sci. 1984 October; 21(4): 399-406. No Abstract Available.
  http://www.ncbi.nlm.nih.gov/entrez/query.fcgi?cmd=Retrieve&db=pubmed&dopt=Abstract&list_uids=6507801

- **Medical Pathology Conference. Headaches and dysphasia in a renal transplant patient.**
  Author(s): Garcia JH, Dismukes WE, Duvall ER.
  Source: Ala J Med Sci. 1981 January; 18(1): 61-7. No Abstract Available.
  http://www.ncbi.nlm.nih.gov/entrez/query.fcgi?cmd=Retrieve&db=pubmed&dopt=Abstract&list_uids=7015899

- **Modern attitudes to the psychology of dysphasia.**
  Author(s): Williams M.
  Source: Br J Disord Commun. 1968 April; 3(1): 60-5. No Abstract Available.
  http://www.ncbi.nlm.nih.gov/entrez/query.fcgi?cmd=Retrieve&db=pubmed&dopt=Abstract&list_uids=5665925

- **Neuropathological abnormalities in developmental dysphasia.**
  Author(s): Cohen M, Campbell R, Yaghmai F.
  Source: Annals of Neurology. 1989 June; 25(6): 567-70.
  http://www.ncbi.nlm.nih.gov/entrez/query.fcgi?cmd=Retrieve&db=pubmed&dopt=Abstract&list_uids=2472772

- **Neuropsychological analysis of a case of crossed dysphasia verified at postmortem.**
  Author(s): Kapur N, Dunkley B.
  Source: Brain and Language. 1984 September; 23(1): 134-47.
  http://www.ncbi.nlm.nih.gov/entrez/query.fcgi?cmd=Retrieve&db=pubmed&dopt=Abstract&list_uids=6206913

- **Nominal dysphasia and the severity of senile dementia.**
  Author(s): Skelton-Robinson M, Jones S.
  Source: The British Journal of Psychiatry; the Journal of Mental Science. 1984 August; 145: 168-71.
  http://www.ncbi.nlm.nih.gov/entrez/query.fcgi?cmd=Retrieve&db=pubmed&dopt=Abstract&list_uids=6466914

- **Nominal dysphasia redux.**
  Author(s): Whiting J.
  Source: Ajr. American Journal of Roentgenology. 1993 May; 160(5): 1146-7.
  http://www.ncbi.nlm.nih.gov/entrez/query.fcgi?cmd=Retrieve&db=pubmed&dopt=Abstract&list_uids=8470597

- **Nominal dysphasia.**
  Author(s): Ronai PM.
  Source: Ajr. American Journal of Roentgenology. 1992 December; 159(6): 1198.
  http://www.ncbi.nlm.nih.gov/entrez/query.fcgi?cmd=Retrieve&db=pubmed&dopt=Abstract&list_uids=1442381

- **Oral dyspraxia in inherited speech and language impairment and acquired dysphasia.**
  Author(s): Alcock KJ, Passingham RE, Watkins KE, Vargha-Khadem F.
  Source: Brain and Language. 2000 October 15; 75(1): 17-33.
  http://www.ncbi.nlm.nih.gov/entrez/query.fcgi?cmd=Retrieve&db=pubmed&dopt=Abstract&list_uids=11023636

- **Origins of paraphasias in deep dysphasia: testing the consequences of a decay impairment to an interactive spreading activation model of lexical retrieval.**
  Author(s): Martin N, Dell GS, Saffran EM, Schwartz MF.
  Source: Brain and Language. 1994 November; 47(4): 609-60.
  http://www.ncbi.nlm.nih.gov/entrez/query.fcgi?cmd=Retrieve&db=pubmed&dopt=Abstract&list_uids=7859057

- **Perception and memory for spatial relations in children with developmental dysphasia.**
  Author(s): Wyke MA, Asso D.
  Source: Neuropsychologia. 1979; 17(2): 231-9.
  http://www.ncbi.nlm.nih.gov/entrez/query.fcgi?cmd=Retrieve&db=pubmed&dopt=Abstract&list_uids=460579

- **Perceptual and acoustical analyses of phonemic paraphasias in nonfluent and fluent dysphasia.**
  Author(s): Holloman AL, Drummond SS.
  Source: Journal of Communication Disorders. 1991 August; 24(4): 301-12.
  http://www.ncbi.nlm.nih.gov/entrez/query.fcgi?cmd=Retrieve&db=pubmed&dopt=Abstract&list_uids=1791217

- **Picture perception, brain damage and dysphasia.**
  Author(s): Reich SS.
  Source: Br J Disord Commun. 1982 December; 17(3): 121-31. No Abstract Available.
  http://www.ncbi.nlm.nih.gov/entrez/query.fcgi?cmd=Retrieve&db=pubmed&dopt=Abstract&list_uids=6190495

- **Pleomorphic adenoma of tongue base causing dysphagia and dysphasia.**
  Author(s): Yoshihara T, Suzuki S.
  Source: The Journal of Laryngology and Otology. 2000 October; 114(10): 793-5. Review.
  http://www.ncbi.nlm.nih.gov/entrez/query.fcgi?cmd=Retrieve&db=pubmed&dopt=Abstract&list_uids=11127155

- **Recovery in deep dysphasia: evidence for a relation between auditory - verbal STM capacity and lexical errors in repetition.**
  Author(s): Martin N, Saffran EM, Dell GS.
  Source: Brain and Language. 1996 January; 52(1): 83-113.
  http://www.ncbi.nlm.nih.gov/entrez/query.fcgi?cmd=Retrieve&db=pubmed&dopt=Abstract&list_uids=8741977

- **Regional brain blood flow in congenital dysphasia: studies with technetium-99m HM-PAO SPECT.**
Author(s): Denays R, Tondeur M, Foulon M, Verstraeten F, Ham H, Piepsz A, Noel P.
Source: Journal of Nuclear Medicine : Official Publication, Society of Nuclear Medicine. 1989 November; 30(11): 1825-9.
http://www.ncbi.nlm.nih.gov/entrez/query.fcgi?cmd=Retrieve&db=pubmed&dopt=Abstract&list_uids=2809746

- **Relation between speech perception and speech production impairment in children with developmental dysphasia.**
Author(s): Tallal P, Stark RE, Curtiss B.
Source: Brain and Language. 1976 April; 3(2): 305-17.
http://www.ncbi.nlm.nih.gov/entrez/query.fcgi?cmd=Retrieve&db=pubmed&dopt=Abstract&list_uids=938935

- **Repeating without semantics: surface dysphasia?**
Author(s): McCarthy RA, Warrington EK.
Source: Neurocase : Case Studies in Neuropsychology, Neuropsychiatry, and Behavioural Neurology. 2001; 7(1): 77-87.
http://www.ncbi.nlm.nih.gov/entrez/query.fcgi?cmd=Retrieve&db=pubmed&dopt=Abstract&list_uids=11239078

- **Resolution of fluent dysphasia following excision of metastatic carcinoma from the arcuate fasciculus.**
Author(s): Tandon PN.
Source: British Journal of Neurosurgery. 1992; 6(4): 389.
http://www.ncbi.nlm.nih.gov/entrez/query.fcgi?cmd=Retrieve&db=pubmed&dopt=Abstract&list_uids=1388837

- **Resolution of fluent dysphasia following excision of metastatic carcinoma from the arcuate fasciculus.**
Author(s): Whittle IR, Fraser DE.
Source: British Journal of Neurosurgery. 1991; 5(6): 647-9.
http://www.ncbi.nlm.nih.gov/entrez/query.fcgi?cmd=Retrieve&db=pubmed&dopt=Abstract&list_uids=1663367

- **Scores on test of gross motor development of children with dysphasia: a pilot study.**
Author(s): Rintala P, Linjala J.
Source: Percept Mot Skills. 2003 December; 97(3 Pt 1): 755-62.
http://www.ncbi.nlm.nih.gov/entrez/query.fcgi?cmd=Retrieve&db=pubmed&dopt=Abstract&list_uids=14738336

- **Sleep EEG and developmental dysphasia.**
Author(s): Picard A, Cheliout Heraut F, Bouskraoui M, Lemoine M, Lacert P, Delattre J.
Source: Developmental Medicine and Child Neurology. 1998 September; 40(9): 595-9.
http://www.ncbi.nlm.nih.gov/entrez/query.fcgi?cmd=Retrieve&db=pubmed&dopt=Abstract&list_uids=9766736

- **'Sleep EEG and developmental dysphasia'.**
  Author(s): Whitehouse W.
  Source: Developmental Medicine and Child Neurology. 1999 February; 41(2): 142-3.
  http://www.ncbi.nlm.nih.gov/entrez/query.fcgi?cmd=Retrieve&db=pubmed&dopt=Abstract&list_uids=10075103

- **Sleep EEG and developmental dysphasia: lack of a consistent relationship with paroxysmal EEG activity during sleep.**
  Author(s): Duvelleroy-Hommet C, Billard C, Lucas B, Gillet P, Barthez MA, Santini JJ, Degiovanni E, Henry F, De Toffol B, Autret A.
  Source: Neuropediatrics. 1995 February; 26(1): 14-8.
  http://www.ncbi.nlm.nih.gov/entrez/query.fcgi?cmd=Retrieve&db=pubmed&dopt=Abstract&list_uids=7540732

- **Some comments on Bishop's annotation "Developmental dysphasia and otitis media".**
  Author(s): Gordon AG.
  Source: Journal of Child Psychology and Psychiatry, and Allied Disciplines. 1988 May; 29(3): 361-8.
  http://www.ncbi.nlm.nih.gov/entrez/query.fcgi?cmd=Retrieve&db=pubmed&dopt=Abstract&list_uids=2458371

- **Status epilepticus presenting as progressive dysphasia.**
  Author(s): Murchison JT, Sellar RJ, Steers AJ.
  Source: Neuroradiology. 1995 August; 37(6): 438-9.
  http://www.ncbi.nlm.nih.gov/entrez/query.fcgi?cmd=Retrieve&db=pubmed&dopt=Abstract&list_uids=7477849

- **Study of unilateral hemisphere performance in children with developmental dysphasia.**
  Author(s): Duvelleroy-Hommet C, Gillet P, Billard C, Loisel ML, Barthez MA, Santini JJ, Autret A.
  Source: Neuropsychologia. 1995 July; 33(7): 823-34.
  http://www.ncbi.nlm.nih.gov/entrez/query.fcgi?cmd=Retrieve&db=pubmed&dopt=Abstract&list_uids=7477810

- **Sulfasalazine induced seizures and dysphasia.**
  Author(s): Hill ME, Gordon C, Situnayake RD, Heath DA.
  Source: The Journal of Rheumatology. 1994 April; 21(4): 748-9.
  http://www.ncbi.nlm.nih.gov/entrez/query.fcgi?cmd=Retrieve&db=pubmed&dopt=Abstract&list_uids=7913503

- **Syndromes in developmental dysphasia and adult aphasia.**
  Author(s): Rapin I, Allen DA.
  Source: Res Publ Assoc Res Nerv Ment Dis. 1988; 66: 57-75. Review.
  http://www.ncbi.nlm.nih.gov/entrez/query.fcgi?cmd=Retrieve&db=pubmed&dopt=Abstract&list_uids=2451853

- **Testing for nominal dysphasia.**
  Author(s): McKenna P, Warrington EK.
  Source: Journal of Neurology, Neurosurgery, and Psychiatry. 1980 September; 43(9): 781-8.
  http://www.ncbi.nlm.nih.gov/entrez/query.fcgi?cmd=Retrieve&db=pubmed&dopt=Abstract&list_uids=7420102

- **The assessment of nominal dysphasia in dementia: the use of reaction-time measures.**
  Author(s): Lawson JS, Barker MG.
  Source: The British Journal of Medical Psychology. 1968 December; 41(4): 411-4.
  http://www.ncbi.nlm.nih.gov/entrez/query.fcgi?cmd=Retrieve&db=pubmed&dopt=Abstract&list_uids=5760127

- **The detection of minimal dysphasia.**
  Author(s): Keenan JS.
  Source: Archives of Physical Medicine and Rehabilitation. 1971 May; 52(5): 227-32.
  http://www.ncbi.nlm.nih.gov/entrez/query.fcgi?cmd=Retrieve&db=pubmed&dopt=Abstract&list_uids=5581034

- **The disturbance of nonverbal functions in dysphasia.**
  Author(s): Smiljkovic P, Filipovic S, Ocic G, Levic Z.
  Source: Neurologija. 1990; 39(4): 251-8.
  http://www.ncbi.nlm.nih.gov/entrez/query.fcgi?cmd=Retrieve&db=pubmed&dopt=Abstract&list_uids=1705313

- **The management of dysphasia in skeletal hyperostosis.**
  Author(s): Akhtar S, O'Flynn PE, Kelly A, Valentine PM.
  Source: The Journal of Laryngology and Otology. 2000 February; 114(2): 154-7.
  http://www.ncbi.nlm.nih.gov/entrez/query.fcgi?cmd=Retrieve&db=pubmed&dopt=Abstract&list_uids=10748839

- **Time to talk: counselling for people with dysphasia.**
  Author(s): Ireland C, Wotton G.
  Source: Disability and Rehabilitation. 1996 November; 18(11): 585-91.
  http://www.ncbi.nlm.nih.gov/entrez/query.fcgi?cmd=Retrieve&db=pubmed&dopt=Abstract&list_uids=9233855

- **Towards a unitary account of access dysphasia: a single case study.**
  Author(s): Cipolotti L, Warrington EK.
  Source: Memory (Hove, England). 1995 September-December; 3(3-4): 309-32.
  http://www.ncbi.nlm.nih.gov/entrez/query.fcgi?cmd=Retrieve&db=pubmed&dopt=Abstract&list_uids=8574868

- **Transient aortic arch syndrome with dysphasia due to ergotism.**
  Author(s): Feneley MP, Morgan JJ, McGrath MA, Egan JD.
  Source: Stroke; a Journal of Cerebral Circulation. 1983 September-October; 14(5): 811-4.
  http://www.ncbi.nlm.nih.gov/entrez/query.fcgi?cmd=Retrieve&db=pubmed&dopt=Abstract&list_uids=6658970

- **Transient expressive (nonfluent) dysphasia after metrizamide myelography.**
  Author(s): Sarno JB.
  Source: Ajnr. American Journal of Neuroradiology. 1985 November-December; 6(6): 945-7.
  http://www.ncbi.nlm.nih.gov/entrez/query.fcgi?cmd=Retrieve&db=pubmed&dopt=Abstract&list_uids=3934934

- **Using fMRI to study recovery from acquired dysphasia.**
  Author(s): Calvert GA, Brammer MJ, Morris RG, Williams SC, King N, Matthews PM.
  Source: Brain and Language. 2000 February 15; 71(3): 391-9.
  http://www.ncbi.nlm.nih.gov/entrez/query.fcgi?cmd=Retrieve&db=pubmed&dopt=Abstract&list_uids=10716869

- **Vertex evoked potentials to tonal, verbal and white noise stimuli in children with developmental dysphasia and dysarthria.**
  Author(s): Novak A.
  Source: Folia Phoniatr (Basel). 1991; 43(5): 215-9. No Abstract Available.
  http://www.ncbi.nlm.nih.gov/entrez/query.fcgi?cmd=Retrieve&db=pubmed&dopt=Abstract&list_uids=1725517

- **Vestibular stimulation, spatial hemineglect and dysphasia, selective effects.**
  Author(s): Vallar G, Papagno C, Rusconi ML, Bisiach E.
  Source: Cortex. 1995 September; 31(3): 589-93.
  http://www.ncbi.nlm.nih.gov/entrez/query.fcgi?cmd=Retrieve&db=pubmed&dopt=Abstract&list_uids=8536486

- **Volunteer and professional treatments of dysphasia after stroke.**
  Author(s): Williams BO, Walker SA.
  Source: British Medical Journal. 1979 September 22; 2(6192): 736.
  http://www.ncbi.nlm.nih.gov/entrez/query.fcgi?cmd=Retrieve&db=pubmed&dopt=Abstract&list_uids=509095

- **Volunteer scheme for dysphasia and allied problems in stroke patients.**
  Author(s): Griffith VE.
  Source: British Medical Journal. 1975 September 13; 3(5984): 633-5.
  http://www.ncbi.nlm.nih.gov/entrez/query.fcgi?cmd=Retrieve&db=pubmed&dopt=Abstract&list_uids=1164643

- **Word retrieval in fluent and nonfluent dysphasia: utilization of pictogram.**
  Author(s): Bracy CB, Drummond SS.
  Source: Journal of Communication Disorders. 1993 June; 26(2): 113-28.
  http://www.ncbi.nlm.nih.gov/entrez/query.fcgi?cmd=Retrieve&db=pubmed&dopt=Abstract&list_uids=8345099

CHAPTER 2. ALTERNATIVE MEDICINE AND DYSPHASIA

Overview

In this chapter, we will begin by introducing you to official information sources on complementary and alternative medicine (CAM) relating to dysphasia. At the conclusion of this chapter, we will provide additional sources.

National Center for Complementary and Alternative Medicine

The National Center for Complementary and Alternative Medicine (NCCAM) of the National Institutes of Health (**http://nccam.nih.gov/**) has created a link to the National Library of Medicine's databases to facilitate research for articles that specifically relate to dysphasia and complementary medicine. To search the database, go to the following Web site: **http://www.nlm.nih.gov/nccam/camonpubmed.html**. Select "CAM on PubMed." Enter "dysphasia" (or synonyms) into the search box. Click "Go." The following references provide information on particular aspects of complementary and alternative medicine that are related to dysphasia:

- **4 case records of acupuncture and moxibustion.**
  Author(s): Du XS.
  Source: J Tradit Chin Med. 1989 December; 9(4): 253-5. No Abstract Available.
  http://www.ncbi.nlm.nih.gov/entrez/query.fcgi?cmd=Retrieve&db=pubmed&dopt=Abstract&list_uids=2483576

- **A comparison of relaxation training and syntax stimulation for chronic nonfluent aphasia.**
  Author(s): Murray LL, Heather Ray A.
  Source: Journal of Communication Disorders. 2001 January-April; 34(1-2): 87-113.
  http://www.ncbi.nlm.nih.gov/entrez/query.fcgi?cmd=Retrieve&db=pubmed&dopt=Abstract&list_uids=11322572

- **A system for the assessment and training of temporal-order discrimination.**
  Author(s): Mates J, von Steinbuchel N, Wittmann M, Treutwein B.

Source: Computer Methods and Programs in Biomedicine. 2001 February; 64(2): 125-131.
http://www.ncbi.nlm.nih.gov/entrez/query.fcgi?cmd=Retrieve&db=pubmed&dopt=Abstract&list_uids=11137195

- **A therapeutic construct for two seven-year-old nonverbal boys.**
  Author(s): Blake JN.
  Source: J Speech Hear Disord. 1969 November; 34(4): 363-9. No Abstract Available.
  http://www.ncbi.nlm.nih.gov/entrez/query.fcgi?cmd=Retrieve&db=pubmed&dopt=Abstract&list_uids=4242484

- **Acquired epileptiform opercular syndrome: a second case report, review of the literature, and comparison to the Landau-Kleffner syndrome.**
  Author(s): Shafrir Y, Prensky AL.
  Source: Epilepsia. 1995 October; 36(10): 1050-7. Review.
  http://www.ncbi.nlm.nih.gov/entrez/query.fcgi?cmd=Retrieve&db=pubmed&dopt=Abstract&list_uids=7555956

- **Acupuncture treatment of wind stroke.**
  Author(s): Hu J.
  Source: J Tradit Chin Med. 1996 December; 16(4): 307-11. No Abstract Available.
  http://www.ncbi.nlm.nih.gov/entrez/query.fcgi?cmd=Retrieve&db=pubmed&dopt=Abstract&list_uids=9389110

- **Adapting role-playing activities with aphasic patients.**
  Author(s): Schlanger PH, Schlanger BB.
  Source: J Speech Hear Disord. 1970 August; 35(3): 229-35. No Abstract Available.
  http://www.ncbi.nlm.nih.gov/entrez/query.fcgi?cmd=Retrieve&db=pubmed&dopt=Abstract&list_uids=5449498

- **Age-related evolution of the contribution of the right hemisphere to language: absence of evidence.**
  Author(s): Nocentini U, Goulet P, Drolet M, Joanette Y.
  Source: The International Journal of Neuroscience. 1999 August; 99(1-4): 59-67.
  http://www.ncbi.nlm.nih.gov/entrez/query.fcgi?cmd=Retrieve&db=pubmed&dopt=Abstract&list_uids=10495196

- **An evaluation of short-term group therapy for people with aphasia.**
  Author(s): Brumfitt SM, Sheeran P.
  Source: Disability and Rehabilitation. 1997 June; 19(6): 221-30.
  http://www.ncbi.nlm.nih.gov/entrez/query.fcgi?cmd=Retrieve&db=pubmed&dopt=Abstract&list_uids=9195139

- **An on-line analysis of syntactic processing in Broca's and Wernicke's aphasia.**
  Author(s): Zurif E, Swinney D, Prather P, Solomon J, Bushell C.
  Source: Brain and Language. 1993 October; 45(3): 448-64.
  http://www.ncbi.nlm.nih.gov/entrez/query.fcgi?cmd=Retrieve&db=pubmed&dopt=Abstract&list_uids=8269334

- **Impairment of auditory perception and language comprehension in dysphasia.**
  Author(s): Tallal P, Newcombe F.

Source: Brain and Language. 1978 January; 5(1): 13-34.
http://www.ncbi.nlm.nih.gov/entrez/query.fcgi?cmd=Retrieve&db=pubmed&dopt=Abstract&list_uids=618565

- **Neurophysiological evidence of auditory channel anomalies in developmental dysphasia.**
  Author(s): Stefanatos GA, Green GG, Ratcliff GG.
  Source: Archives of Neurology. 1989 August; 46(8): 871-5.
  http://www.ncbi.nlm.nih.gov/entrez/query.fcgi?cmd=Retrieve&db=pubmed&dopt=Abstract&list_uids=2757527

- **Rapid resolution following chemotherapy of Broca's dysphasia due to recurrent anaplastic astrocytoma.**
  Author(s): Cole SJ, Fraser DE, Whittle IR.
  Source: British Journal of Neurosurgery. 1994; 8(2): 205-8.
  http://www.ncbi.nlm.nih.gov/entrez/query.fcgi?cmd=Retrieve&db=pubmed&dopt=Abstract&list_uids=7917094

- **The causes of specific developmental language disorder ("development dysphasia").**
  Author(s): Bishop DV.
  Source: Journal of Child Psychology and Psychiatry, and Allied Disciplines. 1987 January; 28(1): 1-8.
  http://www.ncbi.nlm.nih.gov/entrez/query.fcgi?cmd=Retrieve&db=pubmed&dopt=Abstract&list_uids=3558529

Additional Web Resources

A number of additional Web sites offer encyclopedic information covering CAM and related topics. The following is a representative sample:

- Alternative Medicine Foundation, Inc.: **http://www.herbmed.org/**

- AOL: **http://search.aol.com/cat.adp?id=169&layer=&from=subcats**

- Chinese Medicine: **http://www.newcenturynutrition.com/**

- drkoop.com®: **http://www.drkoop.com/InteractiveMedicine/IndexC.html**

- Family Village: **http://www.familyvillage.wisc.edu/med_altn.htm**

- Google: **http://directory.google.com/Top/Health/Alternative/**

- Healthnotes: **http://www.healthnotes.com/**

- MedWebPlus:
  http://medwebplus.com/subject/Alternative_and_Complementary_Medicine

- Open Directory Project: **http://dmoz.org/Health/Alternative/**

- HealthGate: **http://www.tnp.com/**

- WebMD®Health: **http://my.webmd.com/drugs_and_herbs**

- WholeHealthMD.com: **http://www.wholehealthmd.com/reflib/0,1529,00.html**

- Yahoo.com: **http://dir.yahoo.com/Health/Alternative_Medicine/**

The following is a specific Web list relating to dysphasia; please note that any particular subject below may indicate either a therapeutic use, or a contraindication (potential danger), and does not reflect an official recommendation:

- **Chinese Medicine**

    Jixingzi
    Alternative names: Garden Balsam Seed; Semen Impatientis
    Source: Chinese Materia Medica

General References

A good place to find general background information on CAM is the National Library of Medicine. It has prepared within the MEDLINEplus system an information topic page dedicated to complementary and alternative medicine. To access this page, go to the MEDLINEplus site at **http://www.nlm.nih.gov/medlineplus/alternativemedicine.html**. This Web site provides a general overview of various topics and can lead to a number of general sources.

Chapter 3. Patents on Dysphasia

Overview

Patents can be physical innovations (e.g. chemicals, pharmaceuticals, medical equipment) or processes (e.g. treatments or diagnostic procedures). The United States Patent and Trademark Office defines a patent as a grant of a property right to the inventor, issued by the Patent and Trademark Office.[4] Patents, therefore, are intellectual property. For the United States, the term of a new patent is 20 years from the date when the patent application was filed. If the inventor wishes to receive economic benefits, it is likely that the invention will become commercially available within 20 years of the initial filing. It is important to understand, therefore, that an inventor's patent does not indicate that a product or service is or will be commercially available. The patent implies only that the inventor has "the right to exclude others from making, using, offering for sale, or selling" the invention in the United States. While this relates to U.S. patents, similar rules govern foreign patents.

In this chapter, we show you how to locate information on patents and their inventors. If you find a patent that is particularly interesting to you, contact the inventor or the assignee for further information. **IMPORTANT NOTE:** When following the search strategy described below, you may discover <u>non-medical patents</u> that use the generic term "dysphasia" (or a synonym) in their titles. To accurately reflect the results that you might find while conducting research on dysphasia, <u>we have not necessarily excluded non-medical patents</u> in this bibliography.

Patents on Dysphasia

By performing a patent search focusing on dysphasia, you can obtain information such as the title of the invention, the names of the inventor(s), the assignee(s) or the company that owns or controls the patent, a short abstract that summarizes the patent, and a few excerpts from the description of the patent. The abstract of a patent tends to be more technical in nature, while the description is often written for the public. Full patent descriptions contain much more information than is presented here (e.g. claims, references, figures, diagrams, etc.). We will tell you how to obtain this information later in the chapter. The following is an

---

[4]Adapted from the United States Patent and Trademark Office:
http://www.uspto.gov/web/offices/pac/doc/general/whatis.htm.

example of the type of information that you can expect to obtain from a patent search on dysphasia:

- **Single part biocompatible hip-joint socket moorable without cement**

  Inventor(s): Daniel; Peter (Karl Marx Stadt, DD), Krysmann; Waldemar (Karl Marx Stadt, DD), Kurze; Peter (Oberlichtenau, DD), Morgenstern; Rainer (Karl Marx Stadt, DD), Polster; Manfred (Karl Marx Stadt, DD), Rabending; Klaus (Taura, DD), Wehner; Wilfried (Karl Marx Stadt, DD)

  Assignee(s): Technische Universitaet Karl-Marx-Stadt (Karl Marx Stadt, DD)

  Patent Number: 4,801,300

  Date filed: December 23, 1987

  Abstract: The invention relates to a single-part, biocompatible hip-joint socket moorable without cement, which hip-joint socket can be used universally in combination with hip-joint endoprostheses and is especially suitable for the treatment of **dysphasia** hips. The joint socket is made of Ti or Ta metals forming a barrier layer or of alloys thereof and is provided with a perforated flange ring for screwing to the pelvic bone, as well as being provided over its entire surface with specific function characteristic oxide layers containing bioactivators. For the implantation of the hip-joint socket, there are not required any special operating instructions, and additional operations, such as pelvic osteotomies, plasties of the roof of the acetabulum and repeated operations are prevented or minimized.

  Excerpt(s): This invention relates to a single-part biocompatible hip-joint socket moorable without cement for use as an endoprosthesis. Hip-joint sockets for surgical use are made of plastics, preferably polyethylene or metal combined with polyethylene or solid ceramics. Polyethylene used for hip-joint sockets (DE-OS No. 3200340, CH-P648747) in its compactness has a relatively good biocompatibility. It is known, however, that abrasions which are caused by the action of the joint head can be resorbed only with difficulty or not at all by the human body. Thus, there can occur inflammations which can require further operations. In spite of the moorage profiles mounted on the joint socket consisting of polyethylene (CH-P No. 648747) there is attained only an insufficient long-term stabilization.

  Web site: http://www.delphion.com/details?pn=US04801300__

Patent Applications on Dysphasia

As of December 2000, U.S. patent applications are open to public viewing.[5] Applications are patent requests which have yet to be granted. (The process to achieve a patent can take several years.) The following patent applications have been filed since December 2000 relating to dysphasia:

---

[5] This has been a common practice outside the United States prior to December 2000.

- **Systems and methods for treating a mucosal surface**

  Inventor(s): Hedenstrom, John C.; (St. Paul, MN), Jozwiakowski, Michael J.; (Stillwater, MN), Martinez, Mark; (San Francisco, CA), Phares, Kenneth R.; (Chapel Hill, NC), Trofatter, Kenneth JR.; (Minnetonka, MN)

  Correspondence: Finnegan, Henderson, Farabow,; Garrett & Dunner, L.L.P.; 1300 I Street, N.W.; Washington; DC; 20005-3315; US

  Patent Application Number: 20020058674

  Date filed: June 22, 2001

  Abstract: A system for treating a condition associated with a mucosal surface, the system comprising an immune response modifier (IRM) compound chosen from imidazoquinoline amines, imidazopyridine amines, 6,7-fused cycloalkylimidazopyridine amines, imidazonaphthyridine amines, oxazoloquinoline amines, thiazoloquinoline amines, 1,2-bridged imidazoquinoline amines, and pharmaceutically acceptable salts thereof and an applicator device for applying the IRM compound to the mucosal surface. This system of IRM compounds and applicator may be used to treat conditions associated with mucosal surfaces such as cervical **dysphasia** and cervical intraepithelial neoplasia.

  Excerpt(s): This application is a continuation-in-part (CIP) of co-pending application Ser. No. 09/676,339 filed Sep. 29, 2000, which is a continuation of application Ser. No. 09/479,578 filed Jan. 7, 2000 (now U.S. Pat. No. 6,245,776), which claimed priority to application Ser. No. 60/115,253 filed Jan. 8,1999. This application also claims the benefit of priority of the provisional application No. 60/213,420 filed Jun. 22, 2000. In addition, the disclosure of each of the above mentioned applications is incorporated herein by reference. The present invention relates to systems and methods for treating a condition associated with a mucosal surface, such as the vaginal part of the cervix. In particular, the systems and methods may involve an immune response modifier (IRM) compound chosen from imidazoquinoline amines, imidazopyridine amines, 6,7-fused cycloalkylimidazopyridine amines, imidazonaphthyridine amines, oxazoloquinoline amines, thiazoloquinoline amines, 1,2-bridged imidazoquinoline amines, and pharmaceutically acceptable salts thereof. In one optional embodiment, the invention provides systems and methods which are particularly advantageous for topical application to the cervix for treatment of cervical conditions such as cervical dysplasias including dysplasia associated with human papillomavirus (HPV). The present invention is also directed to medicament delivery arrangements and methods of use. Some aspects of the invention are directed to the delivery of a pharmacological agent to a selected location with minimal delivery to regions surrounding the selected location. In some optional embodiments the invention is particularly advantageous for topical delivery of a pharmacological agent to the uterine cervix.

  Web site: http://appft1.uspto.gov/netahtml/PTO/search-bool.html

Keeping Current

In order to stay informed about patents and patent applications dealing with dysphasia, you can access the U.S. Patent Office archive via the Internet at the following Web address: **http://www.uspto.gov/patft/index.html**. You will see two broad options: (1) Issued Patent, and (2) Published Applications. To see a list of issued patents, perform the following steps:

Under "Issued Patents," click "Quick Search." Then, type "dysphasia" (or synonyms) into the "Term 1" box. After clicking on the search button, scroll down to see the various patents which have been granted to date on dysphasia.

You can also use this procedure to view pending patent applications concerning dysphasia. Simply go back to **http://www.uspto.gov/patft/index.html**. Select "Quick Search" under "Published Applications." Then proceed with the steps listed above.

CHAPTER 4. BOOKS ON DYSPHASIA

Overview

This chapter provides bibliographic book references relating to dysphasia. In addition to online booksellers such as **www.amazon.com** and **www.bn.com**, excellent sources for book titles on dysphasia include the Combined Health Information Database and the National Library of Medicine. Your local medical library also may have these titles available for loan.

Book Summaries: Online Booksellers

Commercial Internet-based booksellers, such as Amazon.com and Barnes&Noble.com, offer summaries which have been supplied by each title's publisher. Some summaries also include customer reviews. Your local bookseller may have access to in-house and commercial databases that index all published books (e.g. Books in Print®). **IMPORTANT NOTE:** Online booksellers typically produce search results for medical and non-medical books. When searching for "dysphasia" at online booksellers' Web sites, you may discover non-medical books that use the generic term "dysphasia" (or a synonym) in their titles. The following is indicative of the results you might find when searching for "dysphasia" (sorted alphabetically by title; follow the hyperlink to view more details at Amazon.com):

- **Clinical Aspects of Dysphasia (ACTA Physica Austriaca: Supplementum)** by Martin L. Albert (Other Contributor); ISBN: 0387816178; http://www.amazon.com/exec/obidos/ASIN/0387816178/icongroupinterna

- **Temporal Information Processing in the Nervous System: Special Reference to Dyslexia and Dysphasia (Annals of the New York Academy of Sciences, V)** by Paula Tallal, et al; ISBN: 0897667867; http://www.amazon.com/exec/obidos/ASIN/0897667867/icongroupinterna

- **Understanding Dysphasia (Therapy in Practice Series, No 22)** by Lesley Jordan; ISBN: 0412339102; http://www.amazon.com/exec/obidos/ASIN/0412339102/icongroupinterna

Chapters on Dysphasia

In order to find chapters that specifically relate to dysphasia, an excellent source of abstracts is the Combined Health Information Database. You will need to limit your search to book chapters and dysphasia using the "Detailed Search" option. Go to the following hyperlink: **http://chid.nih.gov/detail/detail.html**. To find book chapters, use the drop boxes at the bottom of the search page where "You may refine your search by." Select the dates and language you prefer, and the format option "Book Chapter." Type "dysphasia" (or synonyms) into the "For these words:" box. The following is a typical result when searching for book chapters on dysphasia:

- **Disorders of Voice, Speech, and Language**

  Source: in Ballenger, J.J.; Snow, J.B., Jr., eds. Otorhinolaryngology: Head and Neck Surgery. 15th ed. Baltimore, MD: Williams and Wilkins. 1996. p. 438-465.

  Contact: Available from Williams and Wilkins. P.O. Box 64686, Baltimore, MD 21264-4786. (800) 638-0672; Fax (800) 447-8438. PRICE: $179.00 plus shipping and handling. ISBN: 0683003151.

  Summary: This chapter, from a medical textbook on otorhinolaryngology, outlines three major categories of communication disorders: disorders of voice, speech, and language. Topics covered include normal voice production, causes of voice disorders, pitch disorders, voice quality disorders, therapy for voice disorders, laryngeal cancer and vocal rehabilitation, disorders of speech, normal speech development in children, articulation disorders, disorders of speech motor control, disorders of fluency (stuttering), disorders of symbolization (language), children with specific language impairment, and aphasia (**dysphasia**) in adults. The authors stress that otolaryngologists must understand communication disorders, not only for consultation with patients, but also as an aid in selecting an appropriate surgical procedure, deciding on other appropriate treatments, or referral. 2 tables. 125 references.

- **Oral Cavity, Pharynx and Esophagus**

  Source: in Strome, M.; Kelly, J.H.; Fried, M.P., eds. Manual of Otolaryngology: Diagnosis and Therapy. 2nd ed. Boston, MA: Little, Brown and Company. 1992. p. 137-171.

  Contact: Available from Little, Brown and Company. 34 Beacon Street, Boston, MA 02108. (800) 759-0190. PRICE: $27.50 plus shipping and handling. ISBN: 0316819689.

  Summary: This chapter, from a reference manual detailing the essentials of otolaryngology and head and neck surgery, discusses the oral cavity, pharynx, and esophagus. Topics covered include oropharyngeal anatomy; physical examination of the pharynx; infectious pharyngitis, including acute bacterial pharyngotonsillitis, diptheria, infectious mononucleosis, Vincent's angina, candidiasis, syphilis, gonococcal pharyngitis, tuberculosis, viral pharyngitis, lingual tonsillitis, nasopharyngitis, and AIDS; noninfectious etiology, including pemphigus, retropharyngeal abscess, parapharyngeal abscess, and submandibular space abscess (Ludwig's angina); allergic edema; tissue hypertrophy, including adenotonsillar hypertrophy, and obstructive sleep apnea; congenital obstruction, including Pierre-Robin syndrome, Thornwald's bursa or nasopharyngeal cyst, and choanal atresia; cysts and neoplasms; **dysphasia;** and esophageal disorders. The manual summarizes the signs and symptoms, diagnosis, and treatment for each disease or disorder. 26 references.

CHAPTER 5. PERIODICALS AND NEWS ON DYSPHASIA

Overview

In this chapter, we suggest a number of news sources and present various periodicals that cover dysphasia.

News Services and Press Releases

One of the simplest ways of tracking press releases on dysphasia is to search the news wires. In the following sample of sources, we will briefly describe how to access each service. These services only post recent news intended for public viewing.

PR Newswire

To access the PR Newswire archive, simply go to **http://www.prnewswire.com/**. Select your country. Type "dysphasia" (or synonyms) into the search box. You will automatically receive information on relevant news releases posted within the last 30 days. The search results are shown by order of relevance.

Reuters Health

The Reuters' Medical News and Health eLine databases can be very useful in exploring news archives relating to dysphasia. While some of the listed articles are free to view, others are available for purchase for a nominal fee. To access this archive, go to **http://www.reutershealth.com/en/index.html** and search by "dysphasia" (or synonyms).

The NIH

Within MEDLINEplus, the NIH has made an agreement with the New York Times Syndicate, the AP News Service, and Reuters to deliver news that can be browsed by the public. Search news releases at **http://www.nlm.nih.gov/medlineplus/alphanews_a.html**. MEDLINEplus allows you to browse across an alphabetical index. Or you can search by date at the following Web page: **http://www.nlm.nih.gov/medlineplus/newsbydate.html**. Often, news items are indexed by MEDLINEplus within its search engine.

Business Wire

Business Wire is similar to PR Newswire. To access this archive, simply go to **http://www.businesswire.com/**. You can scan the news by industry category or company name.

Market Wire

Market Wire is more focused on technology than the other wires. To browse the latest press releases by topic, such as alternative medicine, biotechnology, fitness, healthcare, legal, nutrition, and pharmaceuticals, access Market Wire's Medical/Health channel at **http://www.marketwire.com/mw/release_index?channel=MedicalHealth**. Or simply go to Market Wire's home page at **http://www.marketwire.com/mw/home**, type "dysphasia" (or synonyms) into the search box, and click on "Search News." As this service is technology oriented, you may wish to use it when searching for press releases covering diagnostic procedures or tests.

Search Engines

Medical news is also available in the news sections of commercial Internet search engines. See the health news page at Yahoo (**http://dir.yahoo.com/Health/News_and_Media/**), or you can use this Web site's general news search page at **http://news.yahoo.com/**. Type in "dysphasia" (or synonyms). If you know the name of a company that is relevant to dysphasia, you can go to any stock trading Web site (such as **http://www.etrade.com/**) and search for the company name there. News items across various news sources are reported on indicated hyperlinks. Google offers a similar service at **http://news.google.com/**.

BBC

Covering news from a more European perspective, the British Broadcasting Corporation (BBC) allows the public free access to their news archive located at **http://www.bbc.co.uk/**. Search by "dysphasia" (or synonyms).

Newsletter Articles

Use the Combined Health Information Database, and limit your search criteria to "newsletter articles." Again, you will need to use the "Detailed Search" option. Go directly to the following hyperlink: **http://chid.nih.gov/detail/detail.html**. Go to the bottom of the search page where "You may refine your search by." Select the dates and language that you prefer. For the format option, select "Newsletter Article." Type "dysphasia" (or synonyms) into the "For these words:" box. You should check back periodically with this database as it is updated every three months. The following is a typical result when searching for newsletter articles on dysphasia:

- **Dysphagia: When Swallowing Becomes Difficult, See Your Doctor**

Source: Mayo Clinic Health Letter. 16(8): 4-5. August 1998.

Contact: Available from Mayo Clinic Health Letter. Subscription Services, P.O. Box 53889, Boulder, CO 80322-3889. (800) 333-9037 or (303) 604-1465.

Summary: This newsletter article describes dysphagia, or swallowing difficulties. The article outlines the mechanics of swallowing and describes two categories of swallowing disorders: oropharyngeal **dysphasia,** when a stroke or neuromuscular disorder leaves throat muscles weakened; and esophageal dysphagia, which refers to the sensation of food sticking or getting hung up in the base of the throat or chest. Esophageal dysphagia can be caused by peptic stricture (narrowing of the lower esophagus), tumors, certain muscle problems, diverticulum, and complications of radiation therapy for cancer treatment. The article notes the diagnostic tests that may be used to confirm swallowing problems, including barium x-ray, endoscopy, and manometry. The author reminds readers that treatment options for dysphagia depend on the cause of the disorder, but can include diet therapy, physical therapy, esophageal dilatation, drug therapy, and surgery. One sidebar summarizes the questions that patients should think about before going to see their physician; the answers to these questions will help the physician come to an accurate diagnosis. 1 figure.

Academic Periodicals covering Dysphasia

Numerous periodicals are currently indexed within the National Library of Medicine's PubMed database that are known to publish articles relating to dysphasia. In addition to these sources, you can search for articles covering dysphasia that have been published by any of the periodicals listed in previous chapters. To find the latest studies published, go to **http://www.ncbi.nlm.nih.gov/pubmed**, type the name of the periodical into the search box, and click "Go."

If you want complete details about the historical contents of a journal, you can also visit the following Web site: **http://www.ncbi.nlm.nih.gov/entrez/jrbrowser.cgi**. Here, type in the name of the journal or its abbreviation, and you will receive an index of published articles. At **http://locatorplus.gov/**, you can retrieve more indexing information on medical periodicals (e.g. the name of the publisher). Select the button "Search LOCATORplus." Then type in the name of the journal and select the advanced search option "Journal Title Search."

APPENDICES

APPENDIX A. PHYSICIAN RESOURCES

Overview

In this chapter, we focus on databases and Internet-based guidelines and information resources created or written for a professional audience.

NIH Guidelines

Commonly referred to as "clinical" or "professional" guidelines, the National Institutes of Health publish physician guidelines for the most common diseases. Publications are available at the following by relevant Institute[6]:

- Office of the Director (OD); guidelines consolidated across agencies available at http://www.nih.gov/health/consumer/conkey.htm

- National Institute of General Medical Sciences (NIGMS); fact sheets available at http://www.nigms.nih.gov/news/facts/

- National Library of Medicine (NLM); extensive encyclopedia (A.D.A.M., Inc.) with guidelines: http://www.nlm.nih.gov/medlineplus/healthtopics.html

- National Cancer Institute (NCI); guidelines available at http://www.cancer.gov/cancerinfo/list.aspx?viewid=5f35036e-5497-4d86-8c2c-714a9f7c8d25

- National Eye Institute (NEI); guidelines available at http://www.nei.nih.gov/order/index.htm

- National Heart, Lung, and Blood Institute (NHLBI); guidelines available at http://www.nhlbi.nih.gov/guidelines/index.htm

- National Human Genome Research Institute (NHGRI); research available at http://www.genome.gov/page.cfm?pageID=10000375

- National Institute on Aging (NIA); guidelines available at http://www.nia.nih.gov/health/

---

[6] These publications are typically written by one or more of the various NIH Institutes.

- National Institute on Alcohol Abuse and Alcoholism (NIAAA); guidelines available at http://www.niaaa.nih.gov/publications/publications.htm

- National Institute of Allergy and Infectious Diseases (NIAID); guidelines available at http://www.niaid.nih.gov/publications/

- National Institute of Arthritis and Musculoskeletal and Skin Diseases (NIAMS); fact sheets and guidelines available at http://www.niams.nih.gov/hi/index.htm

- National Institute of Child Health and Human Development (NICHD); guidelines available at http://www.nichd.nih.gov/publications/pubskey.cfm

- National Institute on Deafness and Other Communication Disorders (NIDCD); fact sheets and guidelines at http://www.nidcd.nih.gov/health/

- National Institute of Dental and Craniofacial Research (NIDCR); guidelines available at http://www.nidr.nih.gov/health/

- National Institute of Diabetes and Digestive and Kidney Diseases (NIDDK); guidelines available at http://www.niddk.nih.gov/health/health.htm

- National Institute on Drug Abuse (NIDA); guidelines available at http://www.nida.nih.gov/DrugAbuse.html

- National Institute of Environmental Health Sciences (NIEHS); environmental health information available at http://www.niehs.nih.gov/external/facts.htm

- National Institute of Mental Health (NIMH); guidelines available at http://www.nimh.nih.gov/practitioners/index.cfm

- National Institute of Neurological Disorders and Stroke (NINDS); neurological disorder information pages available at http://www.ninds.nih.gov/health_and_medical/disorder_index.htm

- National Institute of Nursing Research (NINR); publications on selected illnesses at http://www.nih.gov/ninr/news-info/publications.html

- National Institute of Biomedical Imaging and Bioengineering; general information at http://grants.nih.gov/grants/becon/becon_info.htm

- Center for Information Technology (CIT); referrals to other agencies based on keyword searches available at http://kb.nih.gov/www_query_main.asp

- National Center for Complementary and Alternative Medicine (NCCAM); health information available at http://nccam.nih.gov/health/

- National Center for Research Resources (NCRR); various information directories available at http://www.ncrr.nih.gov/publications.asp

- Office of Rare Diseases; various fact sheets available at http://rarediseases.info.nih.gov/html/resources/rep_pubs.html

- Centers for Disease Control and Prevention; various fact sheets on infectious diseases available at http://www.cdc.gov/publications.htm

NIH Databases

In addition to the various Institutes of Health that publish professional guidelines, the NIH has designed a number of databases for professionals.[7] Physician-oriented resources provide a wide variety of information related to the biomedical and health sciences, both past and present. The format of these resources varies. Searchable databases, bibliographic citations, full-text articles (when available), archival collections, and images are all available. The following are referenced by the National Library of Medicine:[8]

- **Bioethics:** Access to published literature on the ethical, legal, and public policy issues surrounding healthcare and biomedical research. This information is provided in conjunction with the Kennedy Institute of Ethics located at Georgetown University, Washington, D.C.: **http://www.nlm.nih.gov/databases/databases_bioethics.html**

- **HIV/AIDS Resources:** Describes various links and databases dedicated to HIV/AIDS research: **http://www.nlm.nih.gov/pubs/factsheets/aidsinfs.html**

- **NLM Online Exhibitions:** Describes "Exhibitions in the History of Medicine": **http://www.nlm.nih.gov/exhibition/exhibition.html**. Additional resources for historical scholarship in medicine: **http://www.nlm.nih.gov/hmd/hmd.html**

- **Biotechnology Information:** Access to public databases. The National Center for Biotechnology Information conducts research in computational biology, develops software tools for analyzing genome data, and disseminates biomedical information for the better understanding of molecular processes affecting human health and disease: **http://www.ncbi.nlm.nih.gov/**

- **Population Information:** The National Library of Medicine provides access to worldwide coverage of population, family planning, and related health issues, including family planning technology and programs, fertility, and population law and policy: **http://www.nlm.nih.gov/databases/databases_population.html**

- **Cancer Information:** Access to cancer-oriented databases: **http://www.nlm.nih.gov/databases/databases_cancer.html**

- **Profiles in Science:** Offering the archival collections of prominent twentieth-century biomedical scientists to the public through modern digital technology: **http://www.profiles.nlm.nih.gov/**

- **Chemical Information:** Provides links to various chemical databases and references: **http://sis.nlm.nih.gov/Chem/ChemMain.html**

- **Clinical Alerts:** Reports the release of findings from the NIH-funded clinical trials where such release could significantly affect morbidity and mortality: **http://www.nlm.nih.gov/databases/alerts/clinical_alerts.html**

- **Space Life Sciences:** Provides links and information to space-based research (including NASA): **http://www.nlm.nih.gov/databases/databases_space.html**

- **MEDLINE:** Bibliographic database covering the fields of medicine, nursing, dentistry, veterinary medicine, the healthcare system, and the pre-clinical sciences: **http://www.nlm.nih.gov/databases/databases_medline.html**

---

[7] Remember, for the general public, the National Library of Medicine recommends the databases referenced in MEDLINE*plus* (**http://medlineplus.gov/** or **http://www.nlm.nih.gov/medlineplus/databases.html**).

[8] See **http://www.nlm.nih.gov/databases/databases.html**.

- **Toxicology and Environmental Health Information (TOXNET):** Databases covering toxicology and environmental health: **http://sis.nlm.nih.gov/Tox/ToxMain.html**

- **Visible Human Interface:** Anatomically detailed, three-dimensional representations of normal male and female human bodies: **http://www.nlm.nih.gov/research/visible/visible_human.html**

The NLM Gateway[9]

The NLM (National Library of Medicine) Gateway is a Web-based system that lets users search simultaneously in multiple retrieval systems at the U.S. National Library of Medicine (NLM). It allows users of NLM services to initiate searches from one Web interface, providing one-stop searching for many of NLM's information resources or databases.[10] To use the NLM Gateway, simply go to the search site at **http://gateway.nlm.nih.gov/gw/Cmd**. Type "dysphasia" (or synonyms) into the search box and click "Search." The results will be presented in a tabular form, indicating the number of references in each database category.

Results Summary

Category	Items Found
Journal Articles	7014
Books / Periodicals / Audio Visual	546
Consumer Health	18
Meeting Abstracts	8
Other Collections	39
Total	7625

HSTAT[11]

HSTAT is a free, Web-based resource that provides access to full-text documents used in healthcare decision-making.[12] These documents include clinical practice guidelines, quick-reference guides for clinicians, consumer health brochures, evidence reports and technology assessments from the Agency for Healthcare Research and Quality (AHRQ), as well as AHRQ's Put Prevention Into Practice.[13] Simply search by "dysphasia" (or synonyms) at the following Web site: **http://text.nlm.nih.gov**.

---

[9] Adapted from NLM: **http://gateway.nlm.nih.gov/gw/Cmd?Overview.x**.

[10] The NLM Gateway is currently being developed by the Lister Hill National Center for Biomedical Communications (LHNCBC) at the National Library of Medicine (NLM) of the National Institutes of Health (NIH).

[11] Adapted from HSTAT: **http://www.nlm.nih.gov/pubs/factsheets/hstat.html**.

[12] The HSTAT URL is **http://hstat.nlm.nih.gov/**.

[13] Other important documents in HSTAT include: the National Institutes of Health (NIH) Consensus Conference Reports and Technology Assessment Reports; the HIV/AIDS Treatment Information Service (ATIS) resource documents; the Substance Abuse and Mental Health Services Administration's Center for Substance Abuse Treatment (SAMHSA/CSAT) Treatment Improvement Protocols (TIP) and Center for Substance Abuse Prevention (SAMHSA/CSAP) Prevention Enhancement Protocols System (PEPS); the Public Health Service (PHS) Preventive Services Task Force's *Guide to Clinical Preventive Services*; the independent, nonfederal Task Force on Community Services' *Guide to Community Preventive Services*; and the Health Technology Advisory Committee (HTAC) of the Minnesota Health Care Commission (MHCC) health technology evaluations.

Coffee Break: Tutorials for Biologists[14]

Coffee Break is a general healthcare site that takes a scientific view of the news and covers recent breakthroughs in biology that may one day assist physicians in developing treatments. Here you will find a collection of short reports on recent biological discoveries. Each report incorporates interactive tutorials that demonstrate how bioinformatics tools are used as a part of the research process. Currently, all Coffee Breaks are written by NCBI staff.[15] Each report is about 400 words and is usually based on a discovery reported in one or more articles from recently published, peer-reviewed literature.[16] This site has new articles every few weeks, so it can be considered an online magazine of sorts. It is intended for general background information. You can access the Coffee Break Web site at the following hyperlink: **http://www.ncbi.nlm.nih.gov/Coffeebreak/.**

Other Commercial Databases

In addition to resources maintained by official agencies, other databases exist that are commercial ventures addressing medical professionals. Here are some examples that may interest you:

- **CliniWeb International:** Index and table of contents to selected clinical information on the Internet; see **http://www.ohsu.edu/cliniweb/.**

- **Medical World Search:** Searches full text from thousands of selected medical sites on the Internet; see **http://www.mwsearch.com/.**

---

[14] Adapted from **http://www.ncbi.nlm.nih.gov/Coffeebreak/Archive/FAQ.html.**

[15] The figure that accompanies each article is frequently supplied by an expert external to NCBI, in which case the source of the figure is cited. The result is an interactive tutorial that tells a biological story.

[16] After a brief introduction that sets the work described into a broader context, the report focuses on how a molecular understanding can provide explanations of observed biology and lead to therapies for diseases. Each vignette is accompanied by a figure and hypertext links that lead to a series of pages that interactively show how NCBI tools and resources are used in the research process.

APPENDIX B. PATIENT RESOURCES

Overview

Official agencies, as well as federally funded institutions supported by national grants, frequently publish a variety of guidelines written with the patient in mind. These are typically called "Fact Sheets" or "Guidelines." They can take the form of a brochure, information kit, pamphlet, or flyer. Often they are only a few pages in length. Since new guidelines on dysphasia can appear at any moment and be published by a number of sources, the best approach to finding guidelines is to systematically scan the Internet-based services that post them.

Patient Guideline Sources

The remainder of this chapter directs you to sources which either publish or can help you find additional guidelines on topics related to dysphasia. Due to space limitations, these sources are listed in a concise manner. Do not hesitate to consult the following sources by either using the Internet hyperlink provided, or, in cases where the contact information is provided, contacting the publisher or author directly.

The National Institutes of Health

The NIH gateway to patients is located at **http://health.nih.gov/**. From this site, you can search across various sources and institutes, a number of which are summarized below.

Topic Pages: MEDLINEplus

The National Library of Medicine has created a vast and patient-oriented healthcare information portal called MEDLINEplus. Within this Internet-based system are "health topic pages" which list links to available materials relevant to dysphasia. To access this system, log on to **http://www.nlm.nih.gov/medlineplus/healthtopics.html**. From there you can either search using the alphabetical index or browse by broad topic areas. Recently, MEDLINEplus listed the following when searched for "dysphasia":

Degenerative Nerve Diseases
http://www.nlm.nih.gov/medlineplus/degenerativenervediseases.html

Neuromuscular Disorders
http://www.nlm.nih.gov/medlineplus/neuromusculardisorders.html

Stroke
http://www.nlm.nih.gov/medlineplus/stroke.html

You may also choose to use the search utility provided by MEDLINEplus at the following Web address: **http://www.nlm.nih.gov/medlineplus/**. Simply type a keyword into the search box and click "Search." This utility is similar to the NIH search utility, with the exception that it only includes materials that are linked within the MEDLINEplus system (mostly patient-oriented information). It also has the disadvantage of generating unstructured results. We recommend, therefore, that you use this method only if you have a very targeted search.

The NIH Search Utility

The NIH search utility allows you to search for documents on over 100 selected Web sites that comprise the NIH-WEB-SPACE. Each of these servers is "crawled" and indexed on an ongoing basis. Your search will produce a list of various documents, all of which will relate in some way to dysphasia. The drawbacks of this approach are that the information is not organized by theme and that the references are often a mix of information for professionals and patients. Nevertheless, a large number of the listed Web sites provide useful background information. We can only recommend this route, therefore, for relatively rare or specific disorders, or when using highly targeted searches. To use the NIH search utility, visit the following Web page: **http://search.nih.gov/index.html**.

Additional Web Sources

A number of Web sites are available to the public that often link to government sites. These can also point you in the direction of essential information. The following is a representative sample:

- AOL: **http://search.aol.com/cat.adp?id=168&layer=&from=subcats**

- Family Village: **http://www.familyvillage.wisc.edu/specific.htm**

- Google: **http://directory.google.com/Top/Health/Conditions_and_Diseases/**

- Med Help International: **http://www.medhelp.org/HealthTopics/A.html**

- Open Directory Project: **http://dmoz.org/Health/Conditions_and_Diseases/**

- Yahoo.com: **http://dir.yahoo.com/Health/Diseases_and_Conditions/**

- WebMD®Health: **http://my.webmd.com/health_topics**

Finding Associations

There are several Internet directories that provide lists of medical associations with information on or resources relating to dysphasia. By consulting all of associations listed in this chapter, you will have nearly exhausted all sources for patient associations concerned with dysphasia.

The National Health Information Center (NHIC)

The National Health Information Center (NHIC) offers a free referral service to help people find organizations that provide information about dysphasia. For more information, see the NHIC's Web site at **http://www.health.gov/NHIC/** or contact an information specialist by calling 1-800-336-4797.

Directory of Health Organizations

The Directory of Health Organizations, provided by the National Library of Medicine Specialized Information Services, is a comprehensive source of information on associations. The Directory of Health Organizations database can be accessed via the Internet at **http://www.sis.nlm.nih.gov/Dir/DirMain.html**. It is composed of two parts: DIRLINE and Health Hotlines.

The DIRLINE database comprises some 10,000 records of organizations, research centers, and government institutes and associations that primarily focus on health and biomedicine. To access DIRLINE directly, go to the following Web site: **http://dirline.nlm.nih.gov/**. Simply type in "dysphasia" (or a synonym), and you will receive information on all relevant organizations listed in the database.

Health Hotlines directs you to toll-free numbers to over 300 organizations. You can access this database directly at **http://www.sis.nlm.nih.gov/hotlines/**. On this page, you are given the option to search by keyword or by browsing the subject list. When you have received your search results, click on the name of the organization for its description and contact information.

The Combined Health Information Database

Another comprehensive source of information on healthcare associations is the Combined Health Information Database. Using the "Detailed Search" option, you will need to limit your search to "Organizations" and "dysphasia". Type the following hyperlink into your Web browser: **http://chid.nih.gov/detail/detail.html**. To find associations, use the drop boxes at the bottom of the search page where "You may refine your search by." For publication date, select "All Years." Then, select your preferred language and the format option "Organization Resource Sheet." Type "dysphasia" (or synonyms) into the "For these words:" box. You should check back periodically with this database since it is updated every three months.

The National Organization for Rare Disorders, Inc.

The National Organization for Rare Disorders, Inc. has prepared a Web site that provides, at no charge, lists of associations organized by health topic. You can access this database at the following Web site: **http://www.rarediseases.org/search/orgsearch.html**. Type "dysphasia" (or a synonym) into the search box, and click "Submit Query."

APPENDIX C. FINDING MEDICAL LIBRARIES

Overview

In this Appendix, we show you how to quickly find a medical library in your area.

Preparation

Your local public library and medical libraries have interlibrary loan programs with the National Library of Medicine (NLM), one of the largest medical collections in the world. According to the NLM, most of the literature in the general and historical collections of the National Library of Medicine is available on interlibrary loan to any library. If you would like to access NLM medical literature, then visit a library in your area that can request the publications for you.[17]

Finding a Local Medical Library

The quickest method to locate medical libraries is to use the Internet-based directory published by the National Network of Libraries of Medicine (NN/LM). This network includes 4626 members and affiliates that provide many services to librarians, health professionals, and the public. To find a library in your area, simply visit **http://nnlm.gov/members/adv.html** or call 1-800-338-7657.

Medical Libraries in the U.S. and Canada

In addition to the NN/LM, the National Library of Medicine (NLM) lists a number of libraries with reference facilities that are open to the public. The following is the NLM's list and includes hyperlinks to each library's Web site. These Web pages can provide information on hours of operation and other restrictions. The list below is a small sample of

---

[17] Adapted from the NLM: **http://www.nlm.nih.gov/psd/cas/interlibrary.html**.

libraries recommended by the National Library of Medicine (sorted alphabetically by name of the U.S. state or Canadian province where the library is located)[18]:

- **Alabama:** Health InfoNet of Jefferson County (Jefferson County Library Cooperative, Lister Hill Library of the Health Sciences), **http://www.uab.edu/infonet/**

- **Alabama:** Richard M. Scrushy Library (American Sports Medicine Institute)

- **Arizona:** Samaritan Regional Medical Center: The Learning Center (Samaritan Health System, Phoenix, Arizona), **http://www.samaritan.edu/library/bannerlibs.htm**

- **California:** Kris Kelly Health Information Center (St. Joseph Health System, Humboldt), **http://www.humboldt1.com/~kkhic/index.html**

- **California:** Community Health Library of Los Gatos, **http://www.healthlib.org/orgresources.html**

- **California:** Consumer Health Program and Services (CHIPS) (County of Los Angeles Public Library, Los Angeles County Harbor-UCLA Medical Center Library) - Carson, CA, **http://www.colapublib.org/services/chips.html**

- **California:** Gateway Health Library (Sutter Gould Medical Foundation)

- **California:** Health Library (Stanford University Medical Center), **http://www-med.stanford.edu/healthlibrary/**

- **California:** Patient Education Resource Center - Health Information and Resources (University of California, San Francisco), **http://sfghdean.ucsf.edu/barnett/PERC/default.asp**

- **California:** Redwood Health Library (Petaluma Health Care District), **http://www.phcd.org/rdwdlib.html**

- **California:** Los Gatos PlaneTree Health Library, **http://planetreesanjose.org/**

- **California:** Sutter Resource Library (Sutter Hospitals Foundation, Sacramento), **http://suttermedicalcenter.org/library/**

- **California:** Health Sciences Libraries (University of California, Davis), **http://www.lib.ucdavis.edu/healthsci/**

- **California:** ValleyCare Health Library & Ryan Comer Cancer Resource Center (ValleyCare Health System, Pleasanton), **http://gaelnet.stmarys-ca.edu/other.libs/gbal/east/vchl.html**

- **California:** Washington Community Health Resource Library (Fremont), **http://www.healthlibrary.org/**

- **Colorado:** William V. Gervasini Memorial Library (Exempla Healthcare), **http://www.saintjosephdenver.org/yourhealth/libraries/**

- **Connecticut:** Hartford Hospital Health Science Libraries (Hartford Hospital), **http://www.harthosp.org/library/**

- **Connecticut:** Healthnet: Connecticut Consumer Health Information Center (University of Connecticut Health Center, Lyman Maynard Stowe Library), **http://library.uchc.edu/departm/hnet/**

---

[18] Abstracted from **http://www.nlm.nih.gov/medlineplus/libraries.html**.

- **Connecticut:** Waterbury Hospital Health Center Library (Waterbury Hospital, Waterbury), **http://www.waterburyhospital.com/library/consumer.shtml**

- **Delaware:** Consumer Health Library (Christiana Care Health System, Eugene du Pont Preventive Medicine & Rehabilitation Institute, Wilmington), **http://www.christianacare.org/health_guide/health_guide_pmri_health_info.cfm**

- **Delaware:** Lewis B. Flinn Library (Delaware Academy of Medicine, Wilmington), **http://www.delamed.org/chls.html**

- **Georgia:** Family Resource Library (Medical College of Georgia, Augusta), **http://cmc.mcg.edu/kids_families/fam_resources/fam_res_lib/frl.htm**

- **Georgia:** Health Resource Center (Medical Center of Central Georgia, Macon), **http://www.mccg.org/hrc/hrchome.asp**

- **Hawaii:** Hawaii Medical Library: Consumer Health Information Service (Hawaii Medical Library, Honolulu), **http://hml.org/CHIS/**

- **Idaho:** DeArmond Consumer Health Library (Kootenai Medical Center, Coeur d'Alene), **http://www.nicon.org/DeArmond/index.htm**

- **Illinois:** Health Learning Center of Northwestern Memorial Hospital (Chicago), **http://www.nmh.org/health_info/hlc.html**

- **Illinois:** Medical Library (OSF Saint Francis Medical Center, Peoria), **http://www.osfsaintfrancis.org/general/library/**

- **Kentucky:** Medical Library - Services for Patients, Families, Students & the Public (Central Baptist Hospital, Lexington), **http://www.centralbap.com/education/community/library.cfm**

- **Kentucky:** University of Kentucky - Health Information Library (Chandler Medical Center, Lexington), **http://www.mc.uky.edu/PatientEd/**

- **Louisiana:** Alton Ochsner Medical Foundation Library (Alton Ochsner Medical Foundation, New Orleans), **http://www.ochsner.org/library/**

- **Louisiana:** Louisiana State University Health Sciences Center Medical Library-Shreveport, **http://lib-sh.lsuhsc.edu/**

- **Maine:** Franklin Memorial Hospital Medical Library (Franklin Memorial Hospital, Farmington), **http://www.fchn.org/fmh/lib.htm**

- **Maine:** Gerrish-True Health Sciences Library (Central Maine Medical Center, Lewiston), **http://www.cmmc.org/library/library.html**

- **Maine:** Hadley Parrot Health Science Library (Eastern Maine Healthcare, Bangor), **http://www.emh.org/hll/hpl/guide.htm**

- **Maine:** Maine Medical Center Library (Maine Medical Center, Portland), **http://www.mmc.org/library/**

- **Maine:** Parkview Hospital (Brunswick), **http://www.parkviewhospital.org/**

- **Maine:** Southern Maine Medical Center Health Sciences Library (Southern Maine Medical Center, Biddeford), **http://www.smmc.org/services/service.php3?choice=10**

- **Maine:** Stephens Memorial Hospital's Health Information Library (Western Maine Health, Norway), **http://www.wmhcc.org/Library/**

- **Manitoba, Canada:** Consumer & Patient Health Information Service (University of Manitoba Libraries), http://www.umanitoba.ca/libraries/units/health/reference/chis.html

- **Manitoba, Canada:** J.W. Crane Memorial Library (Deer Lodge Centre, Winnipeg), http://www.deerlodge.mb.ca/crane_library/about.asp

- **Maryland:** Health Information Center at the Wheaton Regional Library (Montgomery County, Dept. of Public Libraries, Wheaton Regional Library), http://www.mont.lib.md.us/healthinfo/hic.asp

- **Massachusetts:** Baystate Medical Center Library (Baystate Health System), http://www.baystatehealth.com/1024/

- **Massachusetts:** Boston University Medical Center Alumni Medical Library (Boston University Medical Center), http://med-libwww.bu.edu/library/lib.html

- **Massachusetts:** Lowell General Hospital Health Sciences Library (Lowell General Hospital, Lowell), http://www.lowellgeneral.org/library/HomePageLinks/WWW.htm

- **Massachusetts:** Paul E. Woodard Health Sciences Library (New England Baptist Hospital, Boston), http://www.nebh.org/health_lib.asp

- **Massachusetts:** St. Luke's Hospital Health Sciences Library (St. Luke's Hospital, Southcoast Health System, New Bedford), http://www.southcoast.org/library/

- **Massachusetts:** Treadwell Library Consumer Health Reference Center (Massachusetts General Hospital), http://www.mgh.harvard.edu/library/chrcindex.html

- **Massachusetts:** UMass HealthNet (University of Massachusetts Medical School, Worchester), http://healthnet.umassmed.edu/

- **Michigan:** Botsford General Hospital Library - Consumer Health (Botsford General Hospital, Library & Internet Services), http://www.botsfordlibrary.org/consumer.htm

- **Michigan:** Helen DeRoy Medical Library (Providence Hospital and Medical Centers), http://www.providence-hospital.org/library/

- **Michigan:** Marquette General Hospital - Consumer Health Library (Marquette General Hospital, Health Information Center), http://www.mgh.org/center.html

- **Michigan:** Patient Education Resouce Center - University of Michigan Cancer Center (University of Michigan Comprehensive Cancer Center, Ann Arbor), http://www.cancer.med.umich.edu/learn/leares.htm

- **Michigan:** Sladen Library & Center for Health Information Resources - Consumer Health Information (Detroit), http://www.henryford.com/body.cfm?id=39330

- **Montana:** Center for Health Information (St. Patrick Hospital and Health Sciences Center, Missoula)

- **National:** Consumer Health Library Directory (Medical Library Association, Consumer and Patient Health Information Section), http://caphis.mlanet.org/directory/index.html

- **National:** National Network of Libraries of Medicine (National Library of Medicine) - provides library services for health professionals in the United States who do not have access to a medical library, http://nnlm.gov/

- **National:** NN/LM List of Libraries Serving the Public (National Network of Libraries of Medicine), http://nnlm.gov/members/

- **Nevada:** Health Science Library, West Charleston Library (Las Vegas-Clark County Library District, Las Vegas), http://www.lvccld.org/special_collections/medical/index.htm

- **New Hampshire:** Dartmouth Biomedical Libraries (Dartmouth College Library, Hanover), http://www.dartmouth.edu/~biomed/resources.htmld/conshealth.htmld/

- **New Jersey:** Consumer Health Library (Rahway Hospital, Rahway), http://www.rahwayhospital.com/library.htm

- **New Jersey:** Dr. Walter Phillips Health Sciences Library (Englewood Hospital and Medical Center, Englewood), http://www.englewoodhospital.com/links/index.htm

- **New Jersey:** Meland Foundation (Englewood Hospital and Medical Center, Englewood), http://www.geocities.com/ResearchTriangle/9360/

- **New York:** Choices in Health Information (New York Public Library) - NLM Consumer Pilot Project participant, http://www.nypl.org/branch/health/links.html

- **New York:** Health Information Center (Upstate Medical University, State University of New York, Syracuse), http://www.upstate.edu/library/hic/

- **New York:** Health Sciences Library (Long Island Jewish Medical Center, New Hyde Park), http://www.lij.edu/library/library.html

- **New York:** ViaHealth Medical Library (Rochester General Hospital), http://www.nyam.org/library/

- **Ohio:** Consumer Health Library (Akron General Medical Center, Medical & Consumer Health Library), http://www.akrongeneral.org/hwlibrary.htm

- **Oklahoma:** The Health Information Center at Saint Francis Hospital (Saint Francis Health System, Tulsa), http://www.sfh-tulsa.com/services/healthinfo.asp

- **Oregon:** Planetree Health Resource Center (Mid-Columbia Medical Center, The Dalles), http://www.mcmc.net/phrc/

- **Pennsylvania:** Community Health Information Library (Milton S. Hershey Medical Center, Hershey), http://www.hmc.psu.edu/commhealth/

- **Pennsylvania:** Community Health Resource Library (Geisinger Medical Center, Danville), http://www.geisinger.edu/education/commlib.shtml

- **Pennsylvania:** HealthInfo Library (Moses Taylor Hospital, Scranton), http://www.mth.org/healthwellness.html

- **Pennsylvania:** Hopwood Library (University of Pittsburgh, Health Sciences Library System, Pittsburgh), http://www.hsls.pitt.edu/guides/chi/hopwood/index_html

- **Pennsylvania:** Koop Community Health Information Center (College of Physicians of Philadelphia), http://www.collphyphil.org/kooppg1.shtml

- **Pennsylvania:** Learning Resources Center - Medical Library (Susquehanna Health System, Williamsport), http://www.shscares.org/services/lrc/index.asp

- **Pennsylvania:** Medical Library (UPMC Health System, Pittsburgh), http://www.upmc.edu/passavant/library.htm

- **Quebec, Canada:** Medical Library (Montreal General Hospital), http://www.mghlib.mcgill.ca/

- **South Dakota:** Rapid City Regional Hospital Medical Library (Rapid City Regional Hospital), **http://www.rcrh.org/Services/Library/Default.asp**

- **Texas:** Houston HealthWays (Houston Academy of Medicine-Texas Medical Center Library), **http://hhw.library.tmc.edu/**

- **Washington:** Community Health Library (Kittitas Valley Community Hospital), **http://www.kvch.com/**

- **Washington:** Southwest Washington Medical Center Library (Southwest Washington Medical Center, Vancouver), **http://www.swmedicalcenter.com/body.cfm?id=72**

ONLINE GLOSSARIES

The Internet provides access to a number of free-to-use medical dictionaries. The National Library of Medicine has compiled the following list of online dictionaries:

- ADAM Medical Encyclopedia (A.D.A.M., Inc.), comprehensive medical reference: **http://www.nlm.nih.gov/medlineplus/encyclopedia.html**

- MedicineNet.com Medical Dictionary (MedicineNet, Inc.): **http://www.medterms.com/Script/Main/hp.asp**

- Merriam-Webster Medical Dictionary (Inteli-Health, Inc.): **http://www.intelihealth.com/IH/**

- Multilingual Glossary of Technical and Popular Medical Terms in Eight European Languages (European Commission) - Danish, Dutch, English, French, German, Italian, Portuguese, and Spanish: **http://allserv.rug.ac.be/~rvdstich/eugloss/welcome.html**

- On-line Medical Dictionary (CancerWEB): **http://cancerweb.ncl.ac.uk/omd/**

- Rare Diseases Terms (Office of Rare Diseases): **http://ord.aspensys.com/asp/diseases/diseases.asp**

- Technology Glossary (National Library of Medicine) - Health Care Technology: **http://www.nlm.nih.gov/nichsr/ta101/ta10108.htm**

Beyond these, MEDLINEplus contains a very patient-friendly encyclopedia covering every aspect of medicine (licensed from A.D.A.M., Inc.). The ADAM Medical Encyclopedia can be accessed at **http://www.nlm.nih.gov/medlineplus/encyclopedia.html**. ADAM is also available on commercial Web sites such as drkoop.com (**http://www.drkoop.com/**) and Web MD (**http://my.webmd.com/adam/asset/adam_disease_articles/a_to_z/a**).

Online Dictionary Directories

The following are additional online directories compiled by the National Library of Medicine, including a number of specialized medical dictionaries:

- Medical Dictionaries: Medical & Biological (World Health Organization): **http://www.who.int/hlt/virtuallibrary/English/diction.htm#Medical**

- MEL-Michigan Electronic Library List of Online Health and Medical Dictionaries (Michigan Electronic Library): **http://mel.lib.mi.us/health/health-dictionaries.html**

- Patient Education: Glossaries (DMOZ Open Directory Project): **http://dmoz.org/Health/Education/Patient_Education/Glossaries/**

- Web of Online Dictionaries (Bucknell University): **http://www.yourdictionary.com/diction5.html#medicine**

DYSPHASIA DICTIONARY

The definitions below are derived from official public sources, including the National Institutes of Health [NIH] and the European Union [EU].

Aberrant: Wandering or deviating from the usual or normal course. [EU]

Abscess: A localized, circumscribed collection of pus. [NIH]

Acantholysis: Separation of the prickle cells of the stratum spinosum of the epidermis, resulting in atrophy of the prickle cell layer. It is seen in diseases such as pemphigus vulgaris (see pemphigus) and keratosis follicularis. [NIH]

Acoustic: Having to do with sound or hearing. [NIH]

Adaptation: 1. The adjustment of an organism to its environment, or the process by which it enhances such fitness. 2. The normal ability of the eye to adjust itself to variations in the intensity of light; the adjustment to such variations. 3. The decline in the frequency of firing of a neuron, particularly of a receptor, under conditions of constant stimulation. 4. In dentistry, (a) the proper fitting of a denture, (b) the degree of proximity and interlocking of restorative material to a tooth preparation, (c) the exact adjustment of bands to teeth. 5. In microbiology, the adjustment of bacterial physiology to a new environment. [EU]

Adenoma: A benign epithelial tumor with a glandular organization. [NIH]

Adverse Effect: An unwanted side effect of treatment. [NIH]

Airway: A device for securing unobstructed passage of air into and out of the lungs during general anesthesia. [NIH]

Alexia: The inability to recognize or comprehend written or printed words. [NIH]

Algorithms: A procedure consisting of a sequence of algebraic formulas and/or logical steps to calculate or determine a given task. [NIH]

Alkaline: Having the reactions of an alkali. [EU]

Alpha Particles: Positively charged particles composed of two protons and two neutrons, i.e., helium nuclei, emitted during disintegration of very heavy isotopes; a beam of alpha particles or an alpha ray has very strong ionizing power, but weak penetrability. [NIH]

Alternative medicine: Practices not generally recognized by the medical community as standard or conventional medical approaches and used instead of standard treatments. Alternative medicine includes the taking of dietary supplements, megadose vitamins, and herbal preparations; the drinking of special teas; and practices such as massage therapy, magnet therapy, spiritual healing, and meditation. [NIH]

Alveolar Process: The thickest and spongiest part of the maxilla and mandible hollowed out into deep cavities for the teeth. [NIH]

Amygdala: Almond-shaped group of basal nuclei anterior to the inferior horn of the lateral ventricle of the brain, within the temporal lobe. The amygdala is part of the limbic system. [NIH]

Analog: In chemistry, a substance that is similar, but not identical, to another. [NIH]

Anaplasia: Loss of structural differentiation and useful function of neoplastic cells. [NIH]

Anaplastic: A term used to describe cancer cells that divide rapidly and bear little or no resemblance to normal cells. [NIH]

Anatomical: Pertaining to anatomy, or to the structure of the organism. [EU]

Angina: Chest pain that originates in the heart. [NIH]

Anomalies: Birth defects; abnormalities. [NIH]

Antibody: A type of protein made by certain white blood cells in response to a foreign substance (antigen). Each antibody can bind to only a specific antigen. The purpose of this binding is to help destroy the antigen. Antibodies can work in several ways, depending on the nature of the antigen. Some antibodies destroy antigens directly. Others make it easier for white blood cells to destroy the antigen. [NIH]

Antigens: Substances that are recognized by the immune system and induce an immune reaction. [NIH]

Aphasia: A cognitive disorder marked by an impaired ability to comprehend or express language in its written or spoken form. This condition is caused by diseases which affect the language areas of the dominant hemisphere. Clinical features are used to classify the various subtypes of this condition. General categories include receptive, expressive, and mixed forms of aphasia. [NIH]

Apnea: A transient absence of spontaneous respiration. [NIH]

Apraxia: Loss of ability to perform purposeful movements, in the absence of paralysis or sensory disturbance, caused by lesions in the cortex. [NIH]

Aqueous: Having to do with water. [NIH]

Arteries: The vessels carrying blood away from the heart. [NIH]

Articulation: The relationship of two bodies by means of a moveable joint. [NIH]

Articulation Disorders: Disorders of the quality of speech characterized by the substitution, omission, distortion, and addition of phonemes. [NIH]

Aspiration: The act of inhaling. [NIH]

Asterixis: A motor disturbance marked by intermittency of sustained contraction of groups of muscles. [NIH]

Astrocytes: The largest and most numerous neuroglial cells in the brain and spinal cord. Astrocytes (from "star" cells) are irregularly shaped with many long processes, including those with "end feet" which form the glial (limiting) membrane and directly and indirectly contribute to the blood brain barrier. They regulate the extracellular ionic and chemical environment, and "reactive astrocytes" (along with microglia) respond to injury. Astrocytes have high- affinity transmitter uptake systems, voltage-dependent and transmitter-gated ion channels, and can release transmitter, but their role in signaling (as in many other functions) is not well understood. [NIH]

Astrocytoma: A tumor that begins in the brain or spinal cord in small, star-shaped cells called astrocytes. [NIH]

Atrophy: Decrease in the size of a cell, tissue, organ, or multiple organs, associated with a variety of pathological conditions such as abnormal cellular changes, ischemia, malnutrition, or hormonal changes. [NIH]

Atypical: Irregular; not conformable to the type; in microbiology, applied specifically to strains of unusual type. [EU]

Auditory: Pertaining to the sense of hearing. [EU]

Auditory Perception: The process whereby auditory stimuli are selected, organized and interpreted by the organism; includes speech discrimination. [NIH]

Bacterium: Microscopic organism which may have a spherical, rod-like, or spiral unicellular or non-cellular body. Bacteria usually reproduce through asexual processes. [NIH]

Barium: An element of the alkaline earth group of metals. It has an atomic symbol Ba, atomic number 56, and atomic weight 138. All of its acid-soluble salts are poisonous. [NIH]

Base: In chemistry, the nonacid part of a salt; a substance that combines with acids to form salts; a substance that dissociates to give hydroxide ions in aqueous solutions; a substance whose molecule or ion can combine with a proton (hydrogen ion); a substance capable of donating a pair of electrons (to an acid) for the formation of a coordinate covalent bond. [EU]

Benign: Not cancerous; does not invade nearby tissue or spread to other parts of the body. [NIH]

Bile: An emulsifying agent produced in the liver and secreted into the duodenum. Its composition includes bile acids and salts, cholesterol, and electrolytes. It aids digestion of fats in the duodenum. [NIH]

Biotechnology: Body of knowledge related to the use of organisms, cells or cell-derived constituents for the purpose of developing products which are technically, scientifically and clinically useful. Alteration of biologic function at the molecular level (i.e., genetic engineering) is a central focus; laboratory methods used include transfection and cloning technologies, sequence and structure analysis algorithms, computer databases, and gene and protein structure function analysis and prediction. [NIH]

Blister: Visible accumulations of fluid within or beneath the epidermis. [NIH]

Blood vessel: A tube in the body through which blood circulates. Blood vessels include a network of arteries, arterioles, capillaries, venules, and veins. [NIH]

Bolus: A single dose of drug usually injected into a blood vessel over a short period of time. Also called bolus infusion. [NIH]

Bolus infusion: A single dose of drug usually injected into a blood vessel over a short period of time. Also called bolus. [NIH]

Bone Resorption: Bone loss due to osteoclastic activity. [NIH]

Brachytherapy: A collective term for interstitial, intracavity, and surface radiotherapy. It uses small sealed or partly-sealed sources that may be placed on or near the body surface or within a natural body cavity or implanted directly into the tissues. [NIH]

Candidiasis: Infection with a fungus of the genus Candida. It is usually a superficial infection of the moist cutaneous areas of the body, and is generally caused by C. albicans; it most commonly involves the skin (dermatocandidiasis), oral mucous membranes (thrush, def. 1), respiratory tract (bronchocandidiasis), and vagina (vaginitis). Rarely there is a systemic infection or endocarditis. Called also moniliasis, candidosis, oidiomycosis, and formerly blastodendriosis. [EU]

Candidosis: An infection caused by an opportunistic yeasts that tends to proliferate and become pathologic when the environment is favorable and the host resistance is weakened. [NIH]

Carbon Dioxide: A colorless, odorless gas that can be formed by the body and is necessary for the respiration cycle of plants and animals. [NIH]

Carcinoma: Cancer that begins in the skin or in tissues that line or cover internal organs. [NIH]

Case report: A detailed report of the diagnosis, treatment, and follow-up of an individual patient. Case reports also contain some demographic information about the patient (for example, age, gender, ethnic origin). [NIH]

Cell: The individual unit that makes up all of the tissues of the body. All living things are made up of one or more cells. [NIH]

Cell Respiration: The metabolic process of all living cells (animal and plant) in which oxygen is used to provide a source of energy for the cell. [NIH]

Centrifugation: A method of separating organelles or large molecules that relies upon differential sedimentation through a preformed density gradient under the influence of a gravitational field generated in a centrifuge. [NIH]

Cerebral: Of or pertaining of the cerebrum or the brain. [EU]

Cerebral Palsy: Refers to a motor disability caused by a brain dysfunction. [NIH]

Cerebrum: The largest part of the brain. It is divided into two hemispheres, or halves, called the cerebral hemispheres. The cerebrum controls muscle functions of the body and also controls speech, emotions, reading, writing, and learning. [NIH]

Cervical: Relating to the neck, or to the neck of any organ or structure. Cervical lymph nodes are located in the neck; cervical cancer refers to cancer of the uterine cervix, which is the lower, narrow end (the "neck") of the uterus. [NIH]

Cervical intraepithelial neoplasia: CIN. A general term for the growth of abnormal cells on the surface of the cervix. Numbers from 1 to 3 may be used to describe how much of the cervix contains abnormal cells. [NIH]

Cervix: The lower, narrow end of the uterus that forms a canal between the uterus and vagina. [NIH]

Chemotherapy: Treatment with anticancer drugs. [NIH]

Choanal Atresia: Congenital bony or membranous occlusion of one or both choanae, due to failure of the embryonic bucconasal membrane to rupture. [NIH]

Chronic: A disease or condition that persists or progresses over a long period of time. [NIH]

Clinical trial: A research study that tests how well new medical treatments or other interventions work in people. Each study is designed to test new methods of screening, prevention, diagnosis, or treatment of a disease. [NIH]

Cloning: The production of a number of genetically identical individuals; in genetic engineering, a process for the efficient replication of a great number of identical DNA molecules. [NIH]

Cognition: Intellectual or mental process whereby an organism becomes aware of or obtains knowledge. [NIH]

Collagen: A polypeptide substance comprising about one third of the total protein in mammalian organisms. It is the main constituent of skin, connective tissue, and the organic substance of bones and teeth. Different forms of collagen are produced in the body but all consist of three alpha-polypeptide chains arranged in a triple helix. Collagen is differentiated from other fibrous proteins, such as elastin, by the content of proline, hydroxyproline, and hydroxylysine; by the absence of tryptophan; and particularly by the high content of polar groups which are responsible for its swelling properties. [NIH]

Collapse: 1. A state of extreme prostration and depression, with failure of circulation. 2. Abnormal falling in of the walls of any part of organ. [EU]

Communication Disorders: Disorders of verbal and nonverbal communication caused by receptive or expressive language disorders, cognitive dysfunction (e.g., mental retardation), psychiatric conditions, and hearing disorders. [NIH]

Complement: A term originally used to refer to the heat-labile factor in serum that causes immune cytolysis, the lysis of antibody-coated cells, and now referring to the entire functionally related system comprising at least 20 distinct serum proteins that is the effector not only of immune cytolysis but also of other biologic functions. Complement activation occurs by two different sequences, the classic and alternative pathways. The proteins of the classic pathway are termed 'components of complement' and are designated by the symbols C1 through C9. C1 is a calcium-dependent complex of three distinct proteins C1q, C1r and C1s. The proteins of the alternative pathway (collectively referred to as the properdin system) and complement regulatory proteins are known by semisystematic or trivial names. Fragments resulting from proteolytic cleavage of complement proteins are designated with lower-case letter suffixes, e.g., C3a. Inactivated fragments may be designated with the suffix 'i', e.g. C3bi. Activated components or complexes with biological activity are designated by a bar over the symbol e.g. C1 or C4b,2a. The classic pathway is activated by the binding of C1 to classic pathway activators, primarily antigen-antibody complexes containing IgM, IgG1, IgG3; C1q binds to a single IgM molecule or two adjacent IgG molecules. The alternative pathway can be activated by IgA immune complexes and also by nonimmunologic materials including bacterial endotoxins, microbial polysaccharides, and cell walls. Activation of the classic pathway triggers an enzymatic cascade involving C1, C4, C2 and C3; activation of the alternative pathway triggers a cascade involving C3 and factors B, D and P. Both result in the cleavage of C5 and the formation of the membrane attack complex. Complement activation also results in the formation of many biologically active complement fragments that act as anaphylatoxins, opsonins, or chemotactic factors. [EU]

Complementary and alternative medicine: CAM. Forms of treatment that are used in addition to (complementary) or instead of (alternative) standard treatments. These practices are not considered standard medical approaches. CAM includes dietary supplements, megadose vitamins, herbal preparations, special teas, massage therapy, magnet therapy, spiritual healing, and meditation. [NIH]

Complementary medicine: Practices not generally recognized by the medical community as standard or conventional medical approaches and used to enhance or complement the standard treatments. Complementary medicine includes the taking of dietary supplements, megadose vitamins, and herbal preparations; the drinking of special teas; and practices such as massage therapy, magnet therapy, spiritual healing, and meditation. [NIH]

Computational Biology: A field of biology concerned with the development of techniques for the collection and manipulation of biological data, and the use of such data to make biological discoveries or predictions. This field encompasses all computational methods and theories applicable to molecular biology and areas of computer-based techniques for solving biological problems including manipulation of models and datasets. [NIH]

Connective Tissue: Tissue that supports and binds other tissues. It consists of connective tissue cells embedded in a large amount of extracellular matrix. [NIH]

Connective Tissue: Tissue that supports and binds other tissues. It consists of connective tissue cells embedded in a large amount of extracellular matrix. [NIH]

Connective Tissue Cells: A group of cells that includes fibroblasts, cartilage cells, adipocytes, smooth muscle cells, and bone cells. [NIH]

Consciousness: Sense of awareness of self and of the environment. [NIH]

Consultation: A deliberation between two or more physicians concerning the diagnosis and the proper method of treatment in a case. [NIH]

Contraindications: Any factor or sign that it is unwise to pursue a certain kind of action or treatment, e. g. giving a general anesthetic to a person with pneumonia. [NIH]

Contrast medium: A substance that is introduced into or around a structure and, because of the difference in absorption of x-rays by the contrast medium and the surrounding tissues, allows radiographic visualization of the structure. [EU]

Coordination: Muscular or motor regulation or the harmonious cooperation of muscles or groups of muscles, in a complex action or series of actions. [NIH]

Cortex: The outer layer of an organ or other body structure, as distinguished from the internal substance. [EU]

Cortical: Pertaining to or of the nature of a cortex or bark. [EU]

Curative: Tending to overcome disease and promote recovery. [EU]

Cutaneous: Having to do with the skin. [NIH]

Cyst: A sac or capsule filled with fluid. [NIH]

Degenerative: Undergoing degeneration : tending to degenerate; having the character of or involving degeneration; causing or tending to cause degeneration. [EU]

Deglutition: The process or the act of swallowing. [NIH]

Dementia: An acquired organic mental disorder with loss of intellectual abilities of sufficient severity to interfere with social or occupational functioning. The dysfunction is multifaceted and involves memory, behavior, personality, judgment, attention, spatial relations, language, abstract thought, and other executive functions. The intellectual decline is usually progressive, and initially spares the level of consciousness. [NIH]

Diagnostic procedure: A method used to identify a disease. [NIH]

Digestion: The process of breakdown of food for metabolism and use by the body. [NIH]

Direct: 1. Straight; in a straight line. 2. Performed immediately and without the intervention of subsidiary means. [EU]

Discrimination: The act of qualitative and/or quantitative differentiation between two or more stimuli. [NIH]

Diverticulum: A pathological condition manifested as a pouch or sac opening from a tubular or sacular organ. [NIH]

Dominance: In genetics, the full phenotypic expression of a gene in both heterozygotes and homozygotes. [EU]

Drug Interactions: The action of a drug that may affect the activity, metabolism, or toxicity of another drug. [NIH]

Duodenum: The first part of the small intestine. [NIH]

Dysarthria: Imperfect articulation of speech due to disturbances of muscular control which result from damage to the central or peripheral nervous system. [EU]

Dyslexia: Partial alexia in which letters but not words may be read, or in which words may be read but not understood. [NIH]

Dysphagia: Difficulty in swallowing. [EU]

Edema: Excessive amount of watery fluid accumulated in the intercellular spaces, most commonly present in subcutaneous tissue. [NIH]

Elastin: The protein that gives flexibility to tissues. [NIH]

Electromyography: Recording of the changes in electric potential of muscle by means of surface or needle electrodes. [NIH]

Electrons: Stable elementary particles having the smallest known negative charge, present in all elements; also called negatrons. Positively charged electrons are called positrons. The numbers, energies and arrangement of electrons around atomic nuclei determine the chemical identities of elements. Beams of electrons are called cathode rays or beta rays, the latter being a high-energy biproduct of nuclear decay. [NIH]

Encephalitis: Inflammation of the brain due to infection, autoimmune processes, toxins, and other conditions. Viral infections (see encephalitis, viral) are a relatively frequent cause of this condition. [NIH]

Encephalitis, Viral: Inflammation of brain parenchymal tissue as a result of viral infection. Encephalitis may occur as primary or secondary manifestation of Togaviridae infections; Herpesviridae infections; Adenoviridae infections; Flaviviridae infections; Bunyaviridae infections; Picornaviridae infections; Paramyxoviridae infections; Orthomyxoviridae infections; Retroviridae infections; and Arenaviridae infections. [NIH]

Endocarditis: Exudative and proliferative inflammatory alterations of the endocardium, characterized by the presence of vegetations on the surface of the endocardium or in the endocardium itself, and most commonly involving a heart valve, but sometimes affecting the inner lining of the cardiac chambers or the endocardium elsewhere. It may occur as a primary disorder or as a complication of or in association with another disease. [EU]

Endoscopy: Endoscopic examination, therapy or surgery performed on interior parts of the body. [NIH]

Environmental Health: The science of controlling or modifying those conditions, influences, or forces surrounding man which relate to promoting, establishing, and maintaining health. [NIH]

Epidermis: Nonvascular layer of the skin. It is made up, from within outward, of five layers: 1) basal layer (stratum basale epidermidis); 2) spinous layer (stratum spinosum epidermidis); 3) granular layer (stratum granulosum epidermidis); 4) clear layer (stratum lucidum epidermidis); and 5) horny layer (stratum corneum epidermidis). [NIH]

Epilepticus: Repeated and prolonged epileptic seizures without recovery of consciousness between attacks. [NIH]

Epithelial: Refers to the cells that line the internal and external surfaces of the body. [NIH]

Ergot: Cataract due to ergot poisoning caused by eating of rye cereals contaminated by a fungus. [NIH]

Ergotism: Poisoning caused by ingesting ergotized grain or by the misdirected or excessive use of ergot as a medicine. [NIH]

Esophageal: Having to do with the esophagus, the muscular tube through which food passes from the throat to the stomach. [NIH]

Esophageal Motility Disorders: Disorders affecting the motor function of the upper or lower esophageal sphincters, the esophageal body, or a combination of these parts. The failure of the sphincters to maintain a tonic pressure may result in the impeding of the passage of food, regurgitation of food, or reflux of gastric acid into the esophagus. [NIH]

Esophagus: The muscular tube through which food passes from the throat to the stomach. [NIH]

Evoke: The electric response recorded from the cerebral cortex after stimulation of a peripheral sense organ. [NIH]

Expiration: The act of breathing out, or expelling air from the lungs. [EU]

External-beam radiation: Radiation therapy that uses a machine to aim high-energy rays at the cancer. Also called external radiation. [NIH]

Extracellular: Outside a cell or cells. [EU]

Extracellular Matrix: A meshwork-like substance found within the extracellular space and in association with the basement membrane of the cell surface. It promotes cellular proliferation and provides a supporting structure to which cells or cell lysates in culture dishes adhere. [NIH]

Extremity: A limb; an arm or leg (membrum); sometimes applied specifically to a hand or foot. [EU]

Facial: Of or pertaining to the face. [EU]

Family Planning: Programs or services designed to assist the family in controlling reproduction by either improving or diminishing fertility. [NIH]

Febrile: Pertaining to or characterized by fever. [EU]

Fibrosis: Any pathological condition where fibrous connective tissue invades any organ, usually as a consequence of inflammation or other injury. [NIH]

Forearm: The part between the elbow and the wrist. [NIH]

Fungus: A general term used to denote a group of eukaryotic protists, including mushrooms, yeasts, rusts, moulds, smuts, etc., which are characterized by the absence of chlorophyll and by the presence of a rigid cell wall composed of chitin, mannans, and sometimes cellulose. They are usually of simple morphological form or show some reversible cellular specialization, such as the formation of pseudoparenchymatous tissue in the fruiting body of a mushroom. The dimorphic fungi grow, according to environmental conditions, as moulds or yeasts. [EU]

Gamma Rays: Very powerful and penetrating, high-energy electromagnetic radiation of shorter wavelength than that of x-rays. They are emitted by a decaying nucleus, usually between 0.01 and 10 MeV. They are also called nuclear x-rays. [NIH]

Gastric: Having to do with the stomach. [NIH]

Gastric Acid: Hydrochloric acid present in gastric juice. [NIH]

Gastric Juices: Liquids produced in the stomach to help break down food and kill bacteria. [NIH]

Gene: The functional and physical unit of heredity passed from parent to offspring. Genes are pieces of DNA, and most genes contain the information for making a specific protein. [NIH]

Genetics: The biological science that deals with the phenomena and mechanisms of heredity. [NIH]

Gland: An organ that produces and releases one or more substances for use in the body. Some glands produce fluids that affect tissues or organs. Others produce hormones or participate in blood production. [NIH]

Governing Board: The group in which legal authority is vested for the control of health-related institutions and organizations. [NIH]

Grafting: The operation of transfer of tissue from one site to another. [NIH]

Hearing Disorders: Conditions that impair the transmission or perception of auditory impulses and information from the level of the ear to the temporal cortices, including the sensorineural pathways. [NIH]

Hemiparesis: The weakness or paralysis affecting one side of the body. [NIH]

Hemiplegia: Severe or complete loss of motor function on one side of the body. This condition is usually caused by BRAIN DISEASES that are localized to the cerebral hemisphere opposite to the side of weakness. Less frequently, BRAIN STEM lesions; cervical spinal cord diseases; peripheral nervous system diseases; and other conditions may manifest as hemiplegia. The term hemiparesis (see paresis) refers to mild to moderate weakness involving one side of the body. [NIH]

Hemorrhage: Bleeding or escape of blood from a vessel. [NIH]

Hepatitis: Inflammation of the liver and liver disease involving degenerative or necrotic alterations of hepatocytes. [NIH]

Hepatocytes: The main structural component of the liver. They are specialized epithelial cells that are organized into interconnected plates called lobules. [NIH]

Heterozygotes: Having unlike alleles at one or more corresponding loci on homologous chromosomes. [NIH]

Homozygotes: An individual having a homozygous gene pair. [NIH]

Hormonal: Pertaining to or of the nature of a hormone. [EU]

Human papillomavirus: HPV. A virus that causes abnormal tissue growth (warts) and is often associated with some types of cancer. [NIH]

Hydrogen: The first chemical element in the periodic table. It has the atomic symbol H, atomic number 1, and atomic weight 1. It exists, under normal conditions, as a colorless, odorless, tasteless, diatomic gas. Hydrogen ions are protons. Besides the common H1 isotope, hydrogen exists as the stable isotope deuterium and the unstable, radioactive isotope tritium. [NIH]

Hydroxylysine: A hydroxylated derivative of the amino acid lysine that is present in certain collagens. [NIH]

Hydroxyproline: A hydroxylated form of the imino acid proline. A deficiency in ascorbic acid can result in impaired hydroxyproline formation. [NIH]

Hyperostosis: Increase in the mass of bone per unit volume. [NIH]

Hypertrophy: General increase in bulk of a part or organ, not due to tumor formation, nor to an increase in the number of cells. [NIH]

Hypoglycemia: Abnormally low blood sugar [NIH]

Immune response: The activity of the immune system against foreign substances (antigens). [NIH]

Immune system: The organs, cells, and molecules responsible for the recognition and disposal of foreign ("non-self") material which enters the body. [NIH]

Impairment: In the context of health experience, an impairment is any loss or abnormality of psychological, physiological, or anatomical structure or function. [NIH]

Implant radiation: A procedure in which radioactive material sealed in needles, seeds, wires, or catheters is placed directly into or near the tumor. Also called [NIH]

Implantation: The insertion or grafting into the body of biological, living, inert, or radioactive material. [EU]

Infection: 1. Invasion and multiplication of microorganisms in body tissues, which may be clinically unapparent or result in local cellular injury due to competitive metabolism, toxins, intracellular replication, or antigen-antibody response. The infection may remain localized, subclinical, and temporary if the body's defensive mechanisms are effective. A local infection may persist and spread by extension to become an acute, subacute, or chronic clinical infection or disease state. A local infection may also become systemic when the microorganisms gain access to the lymphatic or vascular system. 2. An infectious disease. [EU]

Infectious Mononucleosis: A common, acute infection usually caused by the Epstein-Barr virus (Human herpesvirus 4). There is an increase in mononuclear white blood cells and other atypical lymphocytes, generalized lymphadenopathy, splenomegaly, and occasionally hepatomegaly with hepatitis. [NIH]

Inflammation: A pathological process characterized by injury or destruction of tissues caused by a variety of cytologic and chemical reactions. It is usually manifested by typical signs of pain, heat, redness, swelling, and loss of function. [NIH]

Internal radiation: A procedure in which radioactive material sealed in needles, seeds, wires, or catheters is placed directly into or near the tumor. Also called brachytherapy, implant radiation, or interstitial radiation therapy. [NIH]

Intraepithelial: Within the layer of cells that form the surface or lining of an organ. [NIH]

Ions: An atom or group of atoms that have a positive or negative electric charge due to a gain (negative charge) or loss (positive charge) of one or more electrons. Atoms with a positive charge are known as cations; those with a negative charge are anions. [NIH]

Ischemia: Deficiency of blood in a part, due to functional constriction or actual obstruction of a blood vessel. [EU]

Kb: A measure of the length of DNA fragments, 1 Kb = 1000 base pairs. The largest DNA fragments are up to 50 kilobases long. [NIH]

Language Disorders: Conditions characterized by deficiencies of comprehension or expression of written and spoken forms of language. These include acquired and developmental disorders. [NIH]

Laryngeal: Having to do with the larynx. [NIH]

Larynx: An irregularly shaped, musculocartilaginous tubular structure, lined with mucous membrane, located at the top of the trachea and below the root of the tongue and the hyoid bone. It is the essential sphincter guarding the entrance into the trachea and functioning secondarily as the organ of voice. [NIH]

Lesion: An area of abnormal tissue change. [NIH]

Lip: Either of the two fleshy, full-blooded margins of the mouth. [NIH]

Liver: A large, glandular organ located in the upper abdomen. The liver cleanses the blood and aids in digestion by secreting bile. [NIH]

Localized: Cancer which has not metastasized yet. [NIH]

Lower Esophageal Sphincter: The muscle between the esophagus and stomach. When a person swallows, this muscle relaxes to let food pass from the esophagus to the stomach. It stays closed at other times to keep stomach contents from flowing back into the esophagus. [NIH]

Lymph: The almost colorless fluid that travels through the lymphatic system and carries cells that help fight infection and disease. [NIH]

Lymph node: A rounded mass of lymphatic tissue that is surrounded by a capsule of connective tissue. Also known as a lymph gland. Lymph nodes are spread out along lymphatic vessels and contain many lymphocytes, which filter the lymphatic fluid (lymph). [NIH]

Lymphadenopathy: Disease or swelling of the lymph nodes. [NIH]

Lymphocytes: White blood cells formed in the body's lymphoid tissue. The nucleus is round or ovoid with coarse, irregularly clumped chromatin while the cytoplasm is typically pale blue with azurophilic (if any) granules. Most lymphocytes can be classified as either T or B (with subpopulations of each); those with characteristics of neither major class are called null cells. [NIH]

Malnutrition: A condition caused by not eating enough food or not eating a balanced diet. [NIH]

Mandible: The largest and strongest bone of the face constituting the lower jaw. It supports the lower teeth. [NIH]

Manifest: Being the part or aspect of a phenomenon that is directly observable : concretely expressed in behaviour. [EU]

Manometry: Tests that measure muscle pressure and movements in the GI tract. [NIH]

Medicament: A medicinal substance or agent. [EU]

MEDLINE: An online database of MEDLARS, the computerized bibliographic Medical Literature Analysis and Retrieval System of the National Library of Medicine. [NIH]

Membrane: A very thin layer of tissue that covers a surface. [NIH]

Memory: Complex mental function having four distinct phases: (1) memorizing or learning, (2) retention, (3) recall, and (4) recognition. Clinically, it is usually subdivided into immediate, recent, and remote memory. [NIH]

Mental: Pertaining to the mind; psychic. 2. (L. mentum chin) pertaining to the chin. [EU]

Mental Processes: Conceptual functions or thinking in all its forms. [NIH]

Mental Retardation: Refers to sub-average general intellectual functioning which originated during the developmental period and is associated with impairment in adaptive behavior. [NIH]

Metastasis: The spread of cancer from one part of the body to another. Tumors formed from cells that have spread are called "secondary tumors" and contain cells that are like those in the original (primary) tumor. The plural is metastases. [NIH]

Metastatic: Having to do with metastasis, which is the spread of cancer from one part of the body to another. [NIH]

Metrizamide: A solute for density gradient centrifugation offering higher maximum solution density without the problems of increased viscosity. It is also used as a resorbable, non-ionic contrast medium. [NIH]

Mobility: Capability of movement, of being moved, or of flowing freely. [EU]

Molecular: Of, pertaining to, or composed of molecules : a very small mass of matter. [EU]

Molecule: A chemical made up of two or more atoms. The atoms in a molecule can be the same (an oxygen molecule has two oxygen atoms) or different (a water molecule has two hydrogen atoms and one oxygen atom). Biological molecules, such as proteins and DNA, can be made up of many thousands of atoms. [NIH]

Monoclonal: An antibody produced by culturing a single type of cell. It therefore consists of a single species of immunoglobulin molecules. [NIH]

Mononuclear: A cell with one nucleus. [NIH]

Motility: The ability to move spontaneously. [EU]

Myelography: X-ray visualization of the spinal cord following injection of contrast medium into the spinal arachnoid space. [NIH]

Nasopharyngitis: Inflammation of the nasopharynx. [NIH]

Nasopharynx: The nasal part of the pharynx, lying above the level of the soft palate. [NIH]

Neoplasia: Abnormal and uncontrolled cell growth. [NIH]

Neoplasms: New abnormal growth of tissue. Malignant neoplasms show a greater degree of anaplasia and have the properties of invasion and metastasis, compared to benign neoplasms. [NIH]

Nervous System: The entire nerve apparatus composed of the brain, spinal cord, nerves and ganglia. [NIH]

Neuromuscular: Pertaining to muscles and nerves. [EU]

Neurosyphilis: A late form of syphilis that affects the brain and may lead to dementia and death. [NIH]

Neutrons: Electrically neutral elementary particles found in all atomic nuclei except light hydrogen; the mass is equal to that of the proton and electron combined and they are unstable when isolated from the nucleus, undergoing beta decay. Slow, thermal, epithermal, and fast neutrons refer to the energy levels with which the neutrons are ejected from heavier nuclei during their decay. [NIH]

Nonverbal Communication: Transmission of emotions, ideas, and attitudes between individuals in ways other than the spoken language. [NIH]

Nucleus: A body of specialized protoplasm found in nearly all cells and containing the chromosomes. [NIH]

On-line: A sexually-reproducing population derived from a common parentage. [NIH]

Oral Health: The optimal state of the mouth and normal functioning of the organs of the mouth without evidence of disease. [NIH]

Oral Hygiene: The practice of personal hygiene of the mouth. It includes the maintenance of oral cleanliness, tissue tone, and general preservation of oral health. [NIH]

Otitis: Inflammation of the ear, which may be marked by pain, fever, abnormalities of hearing, hearing loss, tinnitus, and vertigo. [EU]

Otitis Media: Inflammation of the middle ear. [NIH]

Otolaryngology: A surgical specialty concerned with the study and treatment of disorders of the ear, nose, and throat. [NIH]

Otorhinolaryngology: That branch of medicine concerned with medical and surgical treatment of the head and neck, including the ears, nose and throat. [EU]

Oxygen Consumption: The oxygen consumption is determined by calculating the difference between the amount of oxygen inhaled and exhaled. [NIH]

Palliative: 1. Affording relief, but not cure. 2. An alleviating medicine. [EU]

Papillomavirus: A genus of Papovaviridae causing proliferation of the epithelium, which may lead to malignancy. A wide range of animals are infected including humans, chimpanzees, cattle, rabbits, dogs, and horses. [NIH]

Paralysis: Loss of ability to move all or part of the body. [NIH]

Paraparesis: Mild to moderate loss of bilateral lower extremity motor function, which may be a manifestation of spinal cord diseases; peripheral nervous system diseases; muscular diseases; intracranial hypertension; parasagittal brain lesions; and other conditions. [NIH]

Paresis: A general term referring to a mild to moderate degree of muscular weakness, occasionally used as a synonym for paralysis (severe or complete loss of motor function). In the older literature, paresis often referred specifically to paretic neurosyphilis. "General paresis" and "general paralysis" may still carry that connotation. Bilateral lower extremity paresis is referred to as paraparesis. [NIH]

Paroxysmal: Recurring in paroxysms (= spasms or seizures). [EU]

Pathologic: 1. Indicative of or caused by a morbid condition. 2. Pertaining to pathology (= branch of medicine that treats the essential nature of the disease, especially the structural and functional changes in tissues and organs of the body caused by the disease). [EU]

Pelvic: Pertaining to the pelvis. [EU]

Pelvis: The lower part of the abdomen, located between the hip bones. [NIH]

Pemphigus: Group of chronic blistering diseases characterized histologically by acantholysis and blister formation within the epidermis. [NIH]

Pepsin: An enzyme made in the stomach that breaks down proteins. [NIH]

Peptic: Pertaining to pepsin or to digestion; related to the action of gastric juices. [EU]

Perception: The ability quickly and accurately to recognize similarities and differences among presented objects, whether these be pairs of words, pairs of number series, or multiple sets of these or other symbols such as geometric figures. [NIH]

Periodontitis: Inflammation of the periodontal membrane; also called periodontitis simplex. [NIH]

Peripheral Nervous System: The nervous system outside of the brain and spinal cord. The peripheral nervous system has autonomic and somatic divisions. The autonomic nervous system includes the enteric, parasympathetic, and sympathetic subdivisions. The somatic nervous system includes the cranial and spinal nerves and their ganglia and the peripheral sensory receptors. [NIH]

Peripheral Nervous System Diseases: Diseases of the peripheral nerves external to the brain and spinal cord, which includes diseases of the nerve roots, ganglia, plexi, autonomic nerves, sensory nerves, and motor nerves. [NIH]

Pharmacologic: Pertaining to pharmacology or to the properties and reactions of drugs. [EU]

Pharyngitis: Inflammation of the throat. [NIH]

Pharynx: The hollow tube about 5 inches long that starts behind the nose and ends at the top of the trachea (windpipe) and esophagus (the tube that goes to the stomach). [NIH]

Physical Examination: Systematic and thorough inspection of the patient for physical signs of disease or abnormality. [NIH]

Physical Therapy: The restoration of function and the prevention of disability following disease or injury with the use of light, heat, cold, water, electricity, ultrasound, and exercise. [NIH]

Physiologic: Having to do with the functions of the body. When used in the phrase "physiologic age," it refers to an age assigned by general health, as opposed to calendar age. [NIH]

Pilot study: The initial study examining a new method or treatment. [NIH]

Pitch: The subjective awareness of the frequency or spectral distribution of a sound. [NIH]

Plasticity: In an individual or a population, the capacity for adaptation: a) through gene changes (genetic plasticity) or b) through internal physiological modifications in response to changes of environment (physiological plasticity). [NIH]

Pneumonia: Inflammation of the lungs. [NIH]

Polyethylene: A vinyl polymer made from ethylene. It can be branched or linear. Branched or low-density polyethylene is tough and pliable but not to the same degree as linear polyethylene. Linear or high-density polyethylene has a greater hardness and tensile strength. Polyethylene is used in a variety of products, including implants and prostheses. [NIH]

Polypeptide: A peptide which on hydrolysis yields more than two amino acids; called tripeptides, tetrapeptides, etc. according to the number of amino acids contained. [EU]

Practice Guidelines: Directions or principles presenting current or future rules of policy for the health care practitioner to assist him in patient care decisions regarding diagnosis, therapy, or related clinical circumstances. The guidelines may be developed by government agencies at any level, institutions, professional societies, governing boards, or by the convening of expert panels. The guidelines form a basis for the evaluation of all aspects of health care and delivery. [NIH]

Progressive: Advancing; going forward; going from bad to worse; increasing in scope or severity. [EU]

Proline: A non-essential amino acid that is synthesized from glutamic acid. It is an essential component of collagen and is important for proper functioning of joints and tendons. [NIH]

Prospective Studies: Observation of a population for a sufficient number of persons over a sufficient number of years to generate incidence or mortality rates subsequent to the selection of the study group. [NIH]

Protein S: The vitamin K-dependent cofactor of activated protein C. Together with protein C, it inhibits the action of factors VIIIa and Va. A deficiency in protein S can lead to recurrent venous and arterial thrombosis. [NIH]

Proteins: Polymers of amino acids linked by peptide bonds. The specific sequence of amino acids determines the shape and function of the protein. [NIH]

Protons: Stable elementary particles having the smallest known positive charge, found in the nuclei of all elements. The proton mass is less than that of a neutron. A proton is the nucleus of the light hydrogen atom, i.e., the hydrogen ion. [NIH]

Psychiatric: Pertaining to or within the purview of psychiatry. [EU]

Psychiatry: The medical science that deals with the origin, diagnosis, prevention, and treatment of mental disorders. [NIH]

Psychic: Pertaining to the psyche or to the mind; mental. [EU]

Psychology: The science dealing with the study of mental processes and behavior in man and animals. [NIH]

Psychophysics: The science dealing with the correlation of the physical characteristics of a stimulus, e.g., frequency or intensity, with the response to the stimulus, in order to assess the psychologic factors involved in the relationship. [NIH]

Public Policy: A course or method of action selected, usually by a government, from among alternatives to guide and determine present and future decisions. [NIH]

Pulmonary: Relating to the lungs. [NIH]

Pyrexia: A fever, or a febrile condition; abnormal elevation of the body temperature. [EU]

Radiation: Emission or propagation of electromagnetic energy (waves/rays), or the waves/rays themselves; a stream of electromagnetic particles (electrons, neutrons, protons, alpha particles) or a mixture of these. The most common source is the sun. [NIH]

Radiation therapy: The use of high-energy radiation from x-rays, gamma rays, neutrons, and other sources to kill cancer cells and shrink tumors. Radiation may come from a machine outside the body (external-beam radiation therapy), or it may come from radioactive material placed in the body in the area near cancer cells (internal radiation therapy, implant radiation, or brachytherapy). Systemic radiation therapy uses a radioactive substance, such as a radiolabeled monoclonal antibody, that circulates throughout the body. Also called radiotherapy. [NIH]

Radioactive: Giving off radiation. [NIH]

Radiolabeled: Any compound that has been joined with a radioactive substance. [NIH]

Radiotherapy: The use of ionizing radiation to treat malignant neoplasms and other benign conditions. The most common forms of ionizing radiation used as therapy are x-rays, gamma rays, and electrons. A special form of radiotherapy, targeted radiotherapy, links a cytotoxic radionuclide to a molecule that targets the tumor. When this molecule is an antibody or other immunologic molecule, the technique is called radioimmunotherapy. [NIH]

Receptivity: The condition of the reproductive organs of a female flower that permits effective pollination. [NIH]

Redux: Appetite suppressant. [NIH]

Refer: To send or direct for treatment, aid, information, de decision. [NIH]

Reflux: The term used when liquid backs up into the esophagus from the stomach. [NIH]

Regurgitation: A backward flowing, as the casting up of undigested food, or the backward flowing of blood into the heart, or between the chambers of the heart when a valve is incompetent. [EU]

Resected: Surgical removal of part of an organ. [NIH]

Resorption: The loss of substance through physiologic or pathologic means, such as loss of dentin and cementum of a tooth, or of the alveolar process of the mandible or maxilla. [EU]

Respiration: The act of breathing with the lungs, consisting of inspiration, or the taking into the lungs of the ambient air, and of expiration, or the expelling of the modified air which contains more carbon dioxide than the air taken in (Blakiston's Gould Medical Dictionary, 4th ed.). This does not include tissue respiration (= oxygen consumption) or cell respiration (= cell respiration). [NIH]

Role-play: In this method, a conflict is artificially constructed, and the trainee is given a strategic position in it. [NIH]

Salivary: The duct that convey saliva to the mouth. [NIH]

Sclera: The tough white outer coat of the eyeball, covering approximately the posterior five-sixths of its surface, and continuous anteriorly with the cornea and posteriorly with the external sheath of the optic nerve. [EU]

Scleroderma: A chronic disorder marked by hardening and thickening of the skin. Scleroderma can be localized or it can affect the entire body (systemic). [NIH]

Sclerosis: A pathological process consisting of hardening or fibrosis of an anatomical structure, often a vessel or a nerve. [NIH]

Sclerotic: Pertaining to the outer coat of the eye; the sclera; hard, indurated or sclerosed. [NIH]

Screening: Checking for disease when there are no symptoms. [NIH]

Seizures: Clinical or subclinical disturbances of cortical function due to a sudden, abnormal, excessive, and disorganized discharge of brain cells. Clinical manifestations include abnormal motor, sensory and psychic phenomena. Recurrent seizures are usually referred to as epilepsy or "seizure disorder." [NIH]

Semantics: The relationships between symbols and their meanings. [NIH]

Senile: Relating or belonging to old age; characteristic of old age; resulting from infirmity of old age. [NIH]

Side effect: A consequence other than the one(s) for which an agent or measure is used, as the adverse effects produced by a drug, especially on a tissue or organ system other than the one sought to be benefited by its administration. [EU]

Signs and Symptoms: Clinical manifestations that can be either objective when observed by a physician, or subjective when perceived by the patient. [NIH]

Skeletal: Having to do with the skeleton (boney part of the body). [NIH]

Skeleton: The framework that supports the soft tissues of vertebrate animals and protects many of their internal organs. The skeletons of vertebrates are made of bone and/or cartilage. [NIH]

Skull: The skeleton of the head including the bones of the face and the bones enclosing the brain. [NIH]

Sleep apnea: A serious, potentially life-threatening breathing disorder characterized by repeated cessation of breathing due to either collapse of the upper airway during sleep or absence of respiratory effort. [NIH]

Spastic: 1. Of the nature of or characterized by spasms. 2. Hypertonic, so that the muscles are stiff and the movements awkward. 3. A person exhibiting spasticity, such as occurs in spastic paralysis or in cerebral palsy. [EU]

Spasticity: A state of hypertonicity, or increase over the normal tone of a muscle, with heightened deep tendon reflexes. [EU]

Specialist: In medicine, one who concentrates on 1 special branch of medical science. [NIH]

Species: A taxonomic category subordinate to a genus (or subgenus) and superior to a subspecies or variety, composed of individuals possessing common characters distinguishing them from other categories of individuals of the same taxonomic level. In taxonomic nomenclature, species are designated by the genus name followed by a Latin or Latinized adjective or noun. [EU]

Speech Perception: The process whereby an utterance is decoded into a representation in terms of linguistic units (sequences of phonetic segments which combine to form lexical and grammatical morphemes). [NIH]

Sphincter: A ringlike band of muscle fibres that constricts a passage or closes a natural orifice; called also musculus sphincter. [EU]

Spinal cord: The main trunk or bundle of nerves running down the spine through holes in the spinal bone (the vertebrae) from the brain to the level of the lower back. [NIH]

Spinal Cord Diseases: Pathologic conditions which feature spinal cord damage or dysfunction, including disorders involving the meninges and perimeningeal spaces surrounding the spinal cord. Traumatic injuries, vascular diseases, infections, and inflammatory/autoimmune processes may affect the spinal cord. [NIH]

Spirochete: Lyme disease. [NIH]

Splenomegaly: Enlargement of the spleen. [NIH]

Stabilization: The creation of a stable state. [EU]

Stenosis: Narrowing or stricture of a duct or canal. [EU]

Stimulus: That which can elicit or evoke action (response) in a muscle, nerve, gland or other excitable issue, or cause an augmenting action upon any function or metabolic process. [NIH]

Stomach: An organ of digestion situated in the left upper quadrant of the abdomen between the termination of the esophagus and the beginning of the duodenum. [NIH]

Stress: Forcibly exerted influence; pressure. Any condition or situation that causes strain or tension. Stress may be either physical or psychologic, or both. [NIH]

Stricture: The abnormal narrowing of a body opening. Also called stenosis. [NIH]

Stroke: Sudden loss of function of part of the brain because of loss of blood flow. Stroke may be caused by a clot (thrombosis) or rupture (hemorrhage) of a blood vessel to the brain. [NIH]

Subclinical: Without clinical manifestations; said of the early stage(s) of an infection or other disease or abnormality before symptoms and signs become apparent or detectable by clinical examination or laboratory tests, or of a very mild form of an infection or other disease or abnormality. [EU]

Subcutaneous: Beneath the skin. [NIH]

Submandibular: Four to six lymph glands, located between the lower jaw and the submandibular salivary gland. [NIH]

Syphilis: A contagious venereal disease caused by the spirochete Treponema pallidum.

[NIH]

Systemic: Affecting the entire body. [NIH]

Technetium: The first artificially produced element and a radioactive fission product of uranium. The stablest isotope has a mass number 99 and is used diagnostically as a radioactive imaging agent. Technetium has the atomic symbol Tc, atomic number 43, and atomic weight 98.91. [NIH]

Temporal: One of the two irregular bones forming part of the lateral surfaces and base of the skull, and containing the organs of hearing. [NIH]

Thalamic: Cell that reaches the lateral nucleus of amygdala. [NIH]

Therapeutics: The branch of medicine which is concerned with the treatment of diseases, palliative or curative. [NIH]

Thrombosis: The formation or presence of a blood clot inside a blood vessel. [NIH]

Thrush: A disease due to infection with species of fungi of the genus Candida. [NIH]

Tinnitus: Sounds that are perceived in the absence of any external noise source which may take the form of buzzing, ringing, clicking, pulsations, and other noises. Objective tinnitus refers to noises generated from within the ear or adjacent structures that can be heard by other individuals. The term subjective tinnitus is used when the sound is audible only to the affected individual. Tinnitus may occur as a manifestation of cochlear diseases; vestibulocochlear nerve diseases; intracranial hypertension; craniocerebral trauma; and other conditions. [NIH]

Tissue: A group or layer of cells that are alike in type and work together to perform a specific function. [NIH]

Tonal: Based on special tests used for a topographic diagnosis of perceptive deafness (damage of the Corti organ, peripheral or central damage, i. e. the auditive cortex). [NIH]

Tone: 1. The normal degree of vigour and tension; in muscle, the resistance to passive elongation or stretch; tonus. 2. A particular quality of sound or of voice. 3. To make permanent, or to change, the colour of silver stain by chemical treatment, usually with a heavy metal. [EU]

Tonic: 1. Producing and restoring the normal tone. 2. Characterized by continuous tension. 3. A term formerly used for a class of medicinal preparations believed to have the power of restoring normal tone to tissue. [EU]

Tonsillitis: Inflammation of the tonsils, especially the palatine tonsils. It is often caused by a bacterium. Tonsillitis may be acute, chronic, or recurrent. [NIH]

Tonsils: Small masses of lymphoid tissue on either side of the throat. [NIH]

Topical: On the surface of the body. [NIH]

Toxic: Having to do with poison or something harmful to the body. Toxic substances usually cause unwanted side effects. [NIH]

Toxicity: The quality of being poisonous, especially the degree of virulence of a toxic microbe or of a poison. [EU]

Toxicology: The science concerned with the detection, chemical composition, and pharmacologic action of toxic substances or poisons and the treatment and prevention of toxic manifestations. [NIH]

Toxins: Specific, characterizable, poisonous chemicals, often proteins, with specific biological properties, including immunogenicity, produced by microbes, higher plants, or animals. [NIH]

Trachea: The cartilaginous and membranous tube descending from the larynx and branching into the right and left main bronchi. [NIH]

Transfection: The uptake of naked or purified DNA into cells, usually eukaryotic. It is analogous to bacterial transformation. [NIH]

Tryptophan: An essential amino acid that is necessary for normal growth in infants and for nitrogen balance in adults. It is a precursor serotonin and niacin. [NIH]

Tuberculosis: Any of the infectious diseases of man and other animals caused by species of Mycobacterium. [NIH]

Uranium: A radioactive element of the actinide series of metals. It has an atomic symbol U, atomic number 92, and atomic weight 238.03. U-235 is used as the fissionable fuel in nuclear weapons and as fuel in nuclear power reactors. [NIH]

Uterus: The small, hollow, pear-shaped organ in a woman's pelvis. This is the organ in which a fetus develops. Also called the womb. [NIH]

Vagina: The muscular canal extending from the uterus to the exterior of the body. Also called the birth canal. [NIH]

Vaginal: Of or having to do with the vagina, the birth canal. [NIH]

Vaginitis: Inflammation of the vagina characterized by pain and a purulent discharge. [NIH]

Vascular: Pertaining to blood vessels or indicative of a copious blood supply. [EU]

Venereal: Pertaining or related to or transmitted by sexual contact. [EU]

Vertigo: An illusion of movement; a sensation as if the external world were revolving around the patient (objective vertigo) or as if he himself were revolving in space (subjective vertigo). The term is sometimes erroneously used to mean any form of dizziness. [EU]

Veterinary Medicine: The medical science concerned with the prevention, diagnosis, and treatment of diseases in animals. [NIH]

Viral: Pertaining to, caused by, or of the nature of virus. [EU]

Virus: Submicroscopic organism that causes infectious disease. In cancer therapy, some viruses may be made into vaccines that help the body build an immune response to, and kill, tumor cells. [NIH]

Visceral: , from viscus a viscus) pertaining to a viscus. [EU]

Viscosity: A physical property of fluids that determines the internal resistance to shear forces. [EU]

Voice Disorders: Disorders of voice pitch, loudness, or quality. Dysphonia refers to impaired utterance of sounds by the vocal folds. [NIH]

Voice Quality: Voice quality is that component of speech which gives the primary distinction to a given speaker's voice when pitch and loudness are excluded. It involves both phonatory and resonatory characteristics. Some of the descriptions of voice quality are harshness, breathiness and nasality. [NIH]

Warts: Benign epidermal proliferations or tumors; some are viral in origin. [NIH]

White blood cell: A type of cell in the immune system that helps the body fight infection and disease. White blood cells include lymphocytes, granulocytes, macrophages, and others. [NIH]

Windpipe: A rigid tube, 10 cm long, extending from the cricoid cartilage to the upper border of the fifth thoracic vertebra. [NIH]

X-ray: High-energy radiation used in low doses to diagnose diseases and in high doses to treat cancer. [NIH]

INDEX

Printed in the United States
47588LVS00002B/9-18